Emergen
Imaging

Mandip K Heir MBChB PG Dip MedEd FRCR
Specialty Registrar in Radiology
University Hospitals of Leicester NHS Trust
Leicester, UK

Ram Vaidhyanath DMRD DNB FRCR
Consultant Radiologist
University Hospitals of Leicester NHS Trust
Leicester, UK

JP
medical
publishers

© 2013 JP Medical Ltd.

Published by JP Medical Ltd, 83 Victoria Street, London, SW1H 0HW, UK

Tel: +44 (0)20 3170 8910 Fax: +44 (0)20 3008 6180

Email: info@jpmedpub.com Web: www.jpmedpub.com

ISBN: 978-1-907816-56-7

British Library Cataloguing in Publication Data
A catalogue record for this book is available from the British Library

Library of Congress Cataloging in Publication Data
A catalog record for this book is available from the Library of Congress

JP Medical Ltd is a subsidiary of Jaypee Brothers Medical Publishers (P) Ltd, New Delhi, India.

Publisher:	Richard Furn
Development Editor:	Paul Mayhew
Design:	Designers Collective Ltd

Typeset, printed and bound in India.

Foreword

Emergency radiology is a rapidly developing subspecialty, whose practitioners are capable of delivering a varied battery of examinations to the full range of emergency patients and presentations, from neonate to centenarian. Optimum patient care requires not only that the radiologist understands the clinical needs of both patient and referrer, but also that the clinician understands the value, risks and limitations of specific imaging tests. *Pocket Tutor Emergency Imaging* addresses this need for mutual understanding, and is therefore of value both to radiologists and radiographers working in emergency imaging, to clinicians referring their patients to the X-ray department, and to students and trainees.

Taking a system-based approach, this book deals with the common emergency presentations. Key radiological anatomy, types of abnormalities seen and the importance of interpreting the normal result are all presented in a clinical context.

The authors are especially well placed to write this volume. The Leicester Royal Infirmary is one of the United Kingdom's busiest emergency hospitals and the site of one of the country's first dedicated emergency radiology departments. The emergency radiology (ER) department is staffed by specialist trainees 24/7 and forms a pivotal part of our radiology training scheme. The depth of this clinical and educational experience is strongly reflected in the practical and straightforward approach of this book.

The role of emergency radiologists is challenging. They are required to be capable of working under pressure, constantly reprioritising work according to clinical need and continually communicating with patients and referrers to ensure each patient gets the right test/report at the right time. This volume invites you to share this world, and will help you develop your own clinical skills, to the benefit of your patients.

Professor Graham Cherryman
Honorary Consultant Radiologist
University Hospitals of Leicester NHS Trust
Honorary Professor of Radiology, University of Leicester
Leicester, UK

Preface

Pocket Tutor Emergency Imaging is written to help students, trainees and clinicians interpret imaging results when investigating common emergency clinical conditions. It also serves as a guide as to which imaging techniques to request, and when to request them.

The opening chapter explains the principles of emergency imaging and patient safety considerations, including some elementary physics for the common imaging modalities. The next two chapters present the building blocks for understanding normal and abnormal images. Lastly, the clinical chapters are divided into subspecialties, and concisely describe the common emergency conditions, each illustrated by high quality radiological images. A brief reminder of key radiological anatomy is given at the start of each clinical chapter, as a quick reference guide. Clinical insight and guiding principle boxes throughout the text draw upon our own clinical experience in managing these emergency conditions.

Although a pocket-sized book like this cannot be exhaustive, we have aimed to provide comprehensive coverage of the common emergency clinical conditions that a junior doctor will be faced with, in a range of subspecialties. We hope that it serves as a handy learning tool and reliable companion, helping you to manage patients during busy on-call shifts.

Mandip K Heir
Ram Vaidhyanath
September 2012

Contents

Acknowledgements

We wish to thank our colleagues at the University Hospitals of Leicester for their contribution and suggestions. We also wish to express our gratitude to all the staff at JP Medical and in particular to Paul Mayhew, Development Editor, for his unfailing help during the writing of this book.

MH & RV

I would like to thank my husband, Amandeep for his help and support during the writing and production of this book.

MH

To my wife Rajani and our daughter Nivriti, thank you for your encouragement and support.

RV

Dedication

This book is dedicated to the memory of my father Shankaran Ramachandran, who was an embodiment of simplicity and selfless love for his family.

RV

First principles of emergency imaging

1.1 Imaging modalities

Plain radiographs

The discovery of X-rays by German physicist Wilhelm Conrad Roentgen in 1885 has profoundly influenced medical diagnosis and treatment. Radiographs are used in nearly 70% of diagnostic imaging examinations.

Principles

Radiographs are produced when X-rays pass through a part of the body and the resultant image is captured on a film or imaging plate. The image on the film is the result of the interaction of the X-rays with various tissues of the body part imaged. The amount the X-rays penetrate the body tissue is dependent on the density of the tissue. For example, bone, which has a higher density than soft tissue, allows fewer X-rays to pass through it and hence appears 'white', whereas soft tissue allows more X-rays to pass through and appears dark.

Terminology

Radiolucent Permitting the passage of X-rays with little attenuation and hence almost entirely invisible on X-ray and under fluoroscopy.

Radiopacity The property of being relatively resistant to the passage of X-rays.

Advantages
- X-rays can be used to produce an image of most body parts
- Easily available, even by the bedside, in the emergency department and in operating theatres

Disadvantages
- X-rays provide limited information
- Radiation exposure

Guiding principle

The risks posed by the use of radiation in producing radiographs are usually outweighed by the benefits of helping to make the right diagnosis, aiding patient management.

Ultrasound
Principles
Ultrasound is an imaging technique that uses high-frequency sound waves and their echoes. The ultrasound machine transmits high-frequency (1 to 15 megahertz (MHz)) sound pulses into the body using a probe. Some of the sound waves reflect back to the probe, while some travel on further. The reflected waves are detected by the probe and relayed to the machine. The machine calculates the distance from the probe to the tissue using the speed of sound in tissue (1540 m/s) and the time of each echo's return. This is converted into two-dimensional grayscale images.

Colour Doppler Doppler echoes are usually displayed with grayscale brightness corresponding to their intensity. In colour Doppler, echoes are displayed with colours corresponding to the direction of flow that their positive or negative Doppler shifts represent (towards or away from the transducer). The brightness of the colour represents the intensity of the echoes.

Terminology

Anechoic A structure that does not produce any internal echoes.

Hypoechoic A relative term used to describe an area that has decreased brightness of echoes relative to an adjacent structure.

Hyperechoic Also a relative term, used to describe a structure that has increased brightness of echoes relative to an adjacent structure.

Advantages

- Relatively safe
- Inexpensive
- Readily available by the bedside

Disadvantages

- Heavily operator-dependent
- Limited use in examining bones and deep structures of the body (e.g. the retroperitoneum)

Fluoroscopy
Principle

Fluoroscopy is a common technique used to obtain real-time images of moving body parts and internal structures of a patient compared to static radiographic examinations. In the context of emergency imaging, fluoroscopy is mostly used in paediatric patients to look for upper or lower gastrointestinal (GI) obstructions. It is also used for hydrostatic reduction of intussusception.

Computed tomography
Principles

Computed tomography (CT) uses multiple thin beams of X-rays that pass through a desired volume (part of the body being scanned) from multiple angles (usually over 180 degrees). As the X-rays penetrate the body, the X-ray beams will be attenuated, depending on the type of tissue they have travelled through. On the opposite side from where the X-rays originate, there is an array of detectors measuring the amount of X-rays that have travelled through the volume. This allows determination of the attenuation of individual beams as they pass through the volume.

Examination	Equivalent period of natural back-ground radiation	Estimated lifetime additional risk of cancer per examination
Chest, arms, legs, hands, feet Teeth	A few days	Negligible; less than 1 in 1,000,000
Skull, head, neck	A few weeks	Minimal; 1 in 1,000,000 to 1 in 100,000
Hip, spine, abdomen, pelvis CT scan of head	A few months to a year	Very low; 1 in 100,000 to 1 in 10,000
Kidneys and bladder (IVU) CT scan of chest CT scan of abdomen	A few years	Low; 1 in 10,000 to 3 in 1,000

Table 1.1 Radiation risk of undergoing common X-ray, IVU (intravenous urogram) and CT (computed tomography) examinations.

A computer system assigns a Hounsfield unit to each part of the volume based on the attenuation. The Hounsfield unit relates to the composition of the tissue that has been imaged, representing its density. Hounsfield units range from −1000 (air), which is not dense, to +1000 (cortical bone), which is very dense. CT is very good at discriminating between different types of tissue, including soft tissues (such as adipose and muscular tissue), even though they have similar densities.

Terminology

Isodense Having a density similar to that of another or adjacent tissue, e.g. isodense subdural haematoma.

Hypodense Appears less dense than the surrounding tissue, e.g. fat is hypodense when compared to bone on a CT image.

Hyperdense Appears denser than adjacent tissue, e.g. fresh blood is hyperdense.

Advantages
- Relatively inexpensive compared with magnetic resonance imaging (MRI)

- Accurate, three-dimensional data including attenuation information
- Rapid acquisition of data

Disadvantages
- Relatively high amount of ionising radiation per scan
- Subject to artefacts due to patient movement
- Contrast required for certain structures, particularly vessels. Some patients may have an anaphylactic response to intravenous contrast, which may occasionally be fatal

Clinical insight

The **Canadian CT head rule (CCHR)** is a highly sensitive clinical decision rule for use of CT in patients with minor head injuries. Criteria for performing CT head in patients with minor head injury include:

- Glasgow coma scale (GCS) score lower than 15 two hours after injury
- Suspected open or depressed skull fracture
- Sign of basal skull fracture
- Two or more episodes of vomiting
- Age 65 years or older
- Amnesia before impact of 30 minutes or more
- Dangerous mechanism of injury (e.g. high-speed road traffic accident)

MRI

Principles
An MRI scanner applies a strong magnetic field to an area of interest. Hydrogen atoms present in most tissue placed within this field will mostly align parallel to the external magnetic field. As they align they also spin like a spinning top (precess). Electromagnetic radiation or a radio-frequency pulse is then applied to the precessing nuclei. When the electromagnetic field is turned off, the nuclei will return to their original precession around the external magnetic field. This involves two processes: T1 and T2 relaxation. The information is then converted into an image by computers in the MRI scanner.

Terminology
T1-weighted images convey the longitudinal relaxation time of tissues, whereas T2-weighted images depict the transverse relaxation time.

Hyperintense Brighter than adjacent tissue, e.g. water is hyperintense on T2 images and fat is hyperintense on T1 images.

Hypointense Darker than adjacent tissue, e.g. water is hypo-intense on T1 images.

Advantages
- Superb contrast between different soft tissues
- Higher resolution than CT
- No ionising radiation

Clinical insight

Key contraindications for undergoing MR examination include:
- Most types of pacemaker
- Non-compatible aneurysm clips
- Cochlear implants
- Intraocular foreign body

Disadvantages
- As the diameter of the scanner is quite small, patients may feel claustro-phobic
- Longer examination time when compared to CT
- Contraindicated in patients with pacemaker

1.2 Use of contrast media

Body structures with different densities (i.e. on a chest X-ray the difference between the high-density bone and low-density air provides a contrast) are well seen on plain radiographs and CT. However, it is not possible to distinguish structures with similar density or average atomic numbers. In such cases, a contrast medium is used to improve the contrast between different organs, either by changing the density of the organ (e.g. air in the large bowel in colonography) or increasing the attenuation and Hounsfield unit by injecting a substance such as an iodine-containing contrast medium.

Common radiological investigations that involve the use of contrast media include CT, MRI, intravenous urography (IVU), arteriography and GI tract studies. Radiological contrast media are usually water-soluble with only a small percentage in suspension form. The contrast media most commonly used in emergency imaging are administered intravenously (IV).

Contrast administration
When a power injector is used, a 22G or larger needle/cannula 1.25 - 1.5 inch length is preferred for IV contrast injection. It is

Mild	Nausea, warmth, pallor, flushing (these are normal physiological responses to contrast injection and do not require intervention) Cough, headache, dizziness, vomiting, anxiety, altered taste, itching, chills, shaking, sweats, rash	Signs and symptoms appear self-limiting without evidence of progression. Requires observation (15–20 mins) to confirm resolution and/or lack of progression but usually no treatment. Patient reassurance is usually helpful.
Moderate	Severe urticaria, hypotension, bronchospasm, laryngeal oedema	Oral/IM/IV H_1 antihistamine IV fluids – normal saline O_2 through mask Adrenaline 1:1000–0.5 ml IM Beta$_2$ agonist through inhalers
Severe	Laryngeal oedema, profound hypotension, unresponsiveness, convulsions, clinically manifested arrhythmias, cardiopulmonary arrest	**Call for resus team** Suction airway if necessary Elevate legs if hypotensive O_2 through mask Adrenaline 1:1000–0.5 ml IM Diphenhydramine 25–50 mg IV

Table 1.2 Possible reactions to contrast administration and their management.

advisable to obtain a good backflow of blood to test adequate positioning of the needle in the vein. Adequate positioning of the cannula in the vein is then checked again by flushing 10 ml of saline into the vein before delivering the injection of contrast.

Essential information to establish before the administration of IV contrast includes:

- A history of previous contrast reaction
- Asthma
- Renal problems
- Diabetes
- Metformin therapy

Contrast reactions

Adverse reactions to iodinated contrast media are extremely low, but do occur. They are broadly classified as:

- **Minor**: flushing, nausea, vomiting, pruritis, mild rash, arm pain
- **Moderate**: more severe urticaria, facial oedema, hypotension, bronchospasm
- **Severe**: hypotensive shock, laryngeal oedema, convulsions, respiratory and cardiac arrest

Clinical insight

The following patient groups should have their eGFR tested before contrast administration:

- Over 70 years (recent results within 6 weeks of test)
- Under 70 years but with one or more of the following:
  - Renal disease or surgery on the kidneys
  - Diabetes with renal impairment
  - Dehydration
  - Congestive cardiac failure
  - Concurrent use of nephrotoxic drugs

Clinical insight

There is a lack of valid evidence regarding the **incidence of lactic acidosis** following the administration of IV contrast in patients on metformin therapy. There is no need to stop metformin if the eGFR is more than 60 ml/min/1.73 m^2. If the eGFR is less than 60, any decision to stop metformin for 48 hours should be made in consultation with the clinical team.

Renal function

Contrast media can result in acute renal failure, leading to morbidity and mortality. Contrast media are toxic to the renal tubular ceells as well as resulting in renal ischaemia. Therefore, prior to administration of contrast, patient risk factors such as hypertension, diabetes, and pre-existing renal insufficiency need to be determined.

The development of contrast medium-induced nephropathy is low in people with normal renal function, varying from 0% to 5%. Pre-existing renal impairment increases the frequency of this complication. The **estimated glomerular filtration rate** (eGFR) is more sensitive than serum creatinine levels for assessing the state of renal function before administration of contrast media. A guide level of an eGFR below 60 ml/min/1.73 m^2 has been used to indicate renal impairment.

Understanding normal results

2.1 Plain radiographs

During a radiographic examination, the generated X-ray beam passes though the body part to be examined. As the X-rays pass through the body they can be absorbed or scattered (i.e. they are not strong enough to penetrate the body and so scatter off the surface). The degree to which a given tissue absorbs or scatters X-rays is a function of its density. There are four basic radiographic densities that are important: air, fat, soft tissue and bone (**Figures 2.1** and **2.2**).

Air

When X-rays travel through extremely low-density media, such as air (e.g. lung or bowel gas), they are very weakly absorbed, allowing nearly all of the X-rays' energy to 'blacken' the film.

Fat

Fat is just a shade or two lighter than gas, a dark gray, and becomes important in specific locations.

Soft tissue

Soft tissues and solid organs will both absorb and scatter X-rays to some degree, resulting in a 'grayer' shadow.

Bone

Bone (composed of high molecular weight calcium) will appear predominately 'white' depending on the thickness of the bone (thin rib bones scatter less than a thick vertebral body).

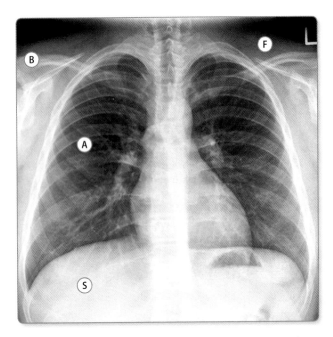

Figure 2.1 A chest radiograph demonstrating (A) air density in the lungs; (B) bone density; (F) fat density; (S) soft tissue density.

2.2 Ultrasound

As the ultrasound (US) beam moves through tissue, it continuously loses energy. This is referred to as attenuation. Several factors contribute to this reduction in energy. One of the most significant is the absorption of the ultrasound energy by the material and its conversion into heat. The rate at which an ultrasound pulse is absorbed generally depends on two factors: (1) the material through which it is passing; and (2) the frequency of the ultrasound. The attenuation (absorption) rate is specified in terms of an attenuation coefficient in the units of decibels per centimetre. The attenuation coefficient of various materials is listed in **Table 2.1**.

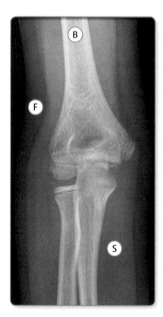

Figure 2.2 A radiograph of the elbow shows (B) bone density; (F) fat density; (S) soft tissue density.

Material	Coefficient (dB/cm/MHz)
Water	0.002
Fat	0.66
Soft tissue (average)	0.9
Muscle (average)	2.0
Air	12.0
Bone	20.0
Lung	40.0

Table 2.1 Approximate attenuation coefficient values for various materials.

Water within the body forms 'windows' through which underlying structures can be easily imaged (e.g. the bladder is a window to scan the uterus in a female patient). Most of the soft tissues of the body have attenuation coefficient values of approximately 1 dB/cm/MHz, with the exception of fat and muscle. The lung has a much higher attenuation rate than either air or soft tissue. Because of this, the normal lung structure is extremely difficult to penetrate with ultrasound. Compared to the soft tissues of the body, bone has a relatively high attenuation rate and, in effect, shields some parts of the body against easy access by ultrasound.

Water
Water or fluid will appear 'dark' or anechoic. This is best seen in the urinary or gall bladders (**Figure 2.3**).

Fat
Fat is brighter than the adjacent soft tissue and its appearance is described as hyperechoic (**Figure 2.4**).

Soft tissue
Soft tissue structures like the liver show a homogenous echogenicity, which can vary from hypoechoic to isoechoic (**Figure 2.5**).

Bone
The cortex of bone is visualised as a thin, well-defined, hyperechoic continuous line (**Figure 2.6**).

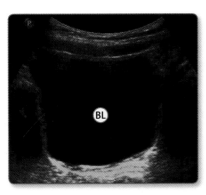

Figure 2.3 An ultrasound of the pelvis. The urinary bladder (**BL**) is uniformly dark or anechoic.

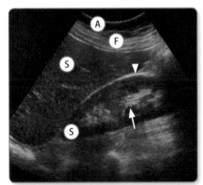

Figure 2.4 An ultrasound of the abdomen. Fat in the perinephric space (arrowhead), in the renal medulla (arrow) and in the subcutaneous fat (F) is echogenic. Compare this with the hypoechoic soft tissue liver and the renal cortex (S) and air overlying the skin (A).

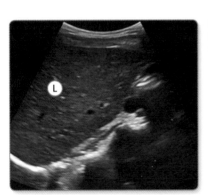

Figure 2.5 Solid organs, such as the liver (L), have a uniform echogenicity.

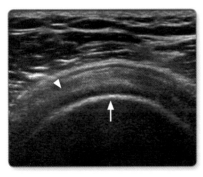

Figure 2.6 An ultrasound of the shoulder. The humeral head is seen as a thin, continuous, echogenic structure (arrow). The supraspinatus muscle (arrowhead) is seen sitting on the bone and has a soft tissue echogenicity.

2.3 CT

The most important output from a computed tomography (CT) scanner is the image itself. Although the reconstructed image represents the linear attenuation coefficient of the part scanned, the actual intensity scale used in CT is the Hounsfield unit (HU). Air has a value of −1000 HU; water has a value of 0 HU; and that of dense bone is +1000 HU. The display monitor uses an 8-bit grayscale representing 256 shades of gray. It is also possible to measure the HU in any area of interest. There are 'windows' which allow images to be reviewed at the most appropriate setting. For example, the bone window setting is best for studying bone abnormality but is not good for showing small differences in attenuation.

Air

The attenuation coefficient of air is nearly zero and will be very dark on CT. Air-containing structures like lungs should be read using the appropriate 'lung' window (**Figure 2.7b**).

Fat

Fat is darker than water but less dark than air (**Figures 2.7**).

Water

Water or fluid density on CT appears less dark than fat (**Figure 2.8**).

Soft tissue

There is a wide range of HU for soft tissue structures. White matter in the brain has a HU of 35 while that of gray matter is 45. It is much higher for solid organs like the liver. All these structures appear gray (**Figure 2.8**).

Bone

Bone ranges in HU from 700 for cancellous bone to over 1000 for dense bone. They appear 'white' on the normal soft tissue window setting but are best demonstrated using the bone window (**Figure 2.9**).

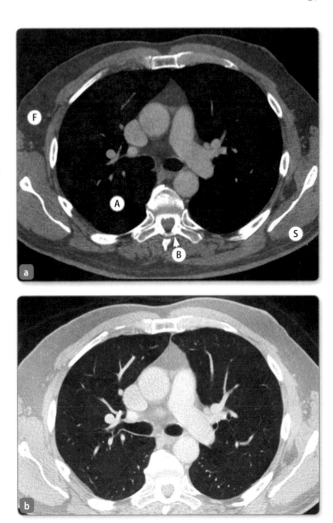

Figure 2.7 (a) A CT of the chest depicting air Ⓐ; bone Ⓑ; fat Ⓕ; and soft tissue Ⓢ densities. (b) A CT of the chest in a lung window setting at the same level as Figure 2.7A. It is important to assess the lung and airway in this window setting.

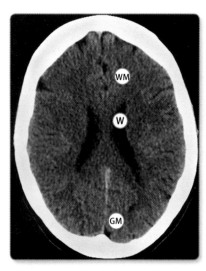

Figure 2.8 A CT of the head at the level of the body of lateral ventricle. cerebrospinal fluid (W) in the ventricle is dark. There is a subtle difference in the density of the white matter (WM) and gray matter (GM).

2.4 MRI

The appearance of various structures on magnetic resonance imaging (MRI) depends upon the imaging sequence. In general, most imaging protocols involve acquiring at least two sequences – T1 and T2 weighted images. In practice, there will be more sequences obtained, depending on the part examined and the clinical question to be answered.

Structure	T1 sequence (Figure 2.10)	T2 sequence (Figure 2.11)
Water	Hypointense (dark)	Hyperintense (bright)
Fat	Hyperintense	Less hyperintense
Soft tissue	Hypo- to iso- intense	Hypo- to iso- intense
Cortical bone	No signal (dark)	No signal (dark)
Medullary bone	Hyperintense	Less hyperintense
Air	Hypointense (dark)	Hypointense (dark)

Table 2.2 The appearance of different structures on T1 and T2 weighted MRI.

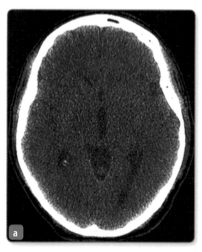

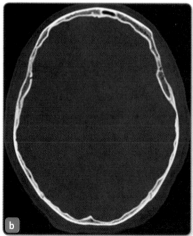

Figure 2.9 (a) A CT of the head in a soft tissue window setting. This is not adequate to assess bone injury. (b) A CT of the head in a bone window setting highlights the bony architecture of the calvarium.

It is important to be familiar with the MR appearances of various structures on both T1 and T2 weighted images. This is summarised in **Table 2.2**.

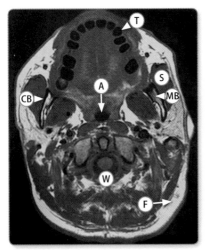

Figure 2.10 A T1 weighted image of the neck at the level of the oropharynx. Air Ⓐ is dark; cerebrospinal fluid around the spinal cord Ⓦ is also dark or hypointense; fat Ⓕ is bright or hyperintense and soft tissue Ⓢ is hypointense; cortical bone ⒸⓂ of mandible is hypointense whereas the medullary bone ⓂⒷ containing fat is hyperintense; denser 'bony' structures like tooth Ⓣ are also hypointense.

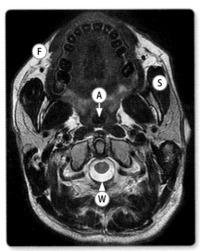

Figure 2.11 A T2 weighted image of the neck at the same level as in figure 2.10. On this sequence, water Ⓦ or fluid is bright or hyperintense; air Ⓐ and soft tissue Ⓢ show little change in signal intensity. Fat Ⓕ remains hyperintense.

Recognising abnormalities

3.1 Fractures

Fractures can occur due to trauma, an underlying pathology or a metabolic problem.

Traumatic fracture

Trauma is the most common cause of a fracture and results from a large force being applied on a normal bone.

X-ray

On plain radiographs, traumatic fractures can be classified as complete or incomplete. Fractures involving both cortices are called complete, whereas fractures that do not extend all the way across the bone are termed incomplete (e.g. greenstick). Complete fractures can be:

- Transverse
- Oblique
- Spiral
- Comminuted (**Figure 3.1**)
- Avulsion (**Figure 3.1**).

CT

Computed tomography (CT) is not the initial imaging modality of choice to assess appendicular bone trauma but is often used for axial skeletal injuries. CT is useful in the assessment of occult appendicular bone injury and to assess possible complications, especially before surgery.

Pathological fractures

Pathological fractures occur in a bone weakened by an underlying process like metastasis, a primary bone tumour, infection or

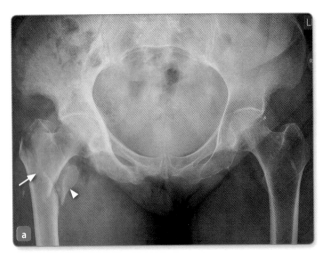

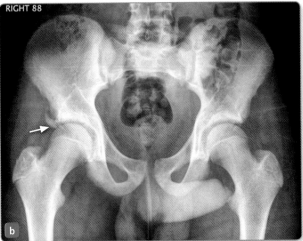

Figure 3.1 Complete fractures. (a) An anteroposterior (AP) pelvic X-ray demonstrating a comminuted fracture of the right neck of femur (arrow) with avulsion of the lesser trochanter (arrowhead). (b) An AP pelvic X-ray demonstrating an avulsion fracture of the right anterior inferior iliac spine at the origin of the rectus femoris muscle (arrow).

metabolic bone disease (**Figure 3.2**). The fracture results from a force insufficient to fracture normal bone.

X-ray

Pathological fractures tend to be oriented transversely in the long bones. Apart from metastatic and primary bone lesions, a diffuse process (like Paget's disease) can also cause pathological fractures.

CT

Pathological fractures are usually demonstrated on CT when performed in the context of staging primary cancer or in the search for an unknown primary cancer. CT is more likely to demonstrate pathological fractures in the spine secondary to metastatic disease.

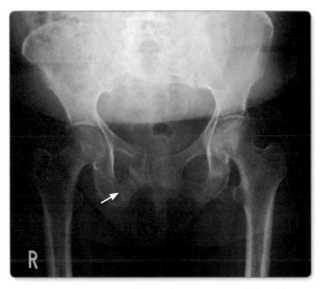

Figure 3.2 An anteroposterior pelvic X-ray demonstrating a pathological fracture of the right inferior pubic ramus through underlying sclerotic bone (arrow).

3.2 Inflammation and abscess

Inflammation is a pathological process characterised by injury or the destruction of tissues caused by a variety of cytological and chemical reactions.

Pathophysiology

The acute response to tissue injury occurs in the microcirculation at the site of the injury. Chemical mediators released at the site cause smooth muscle vasodilation and increased capillary permeability. This results in contrast enhancement of an inflammatory process on CT imaging. Protein-rich fluid then exudes from capillaries into the interstitial space. On ultrasound, CT and magnetic resonance imaging (MRI) this fluid will be seen as a localised collection due to the inflammatory process. Clinical signs of an underlying inflammatory process are redness, swelling, pain, increased temperature at the site of tissue injury and loss of function.

Resolution is the usual outcome of acute inflammation; however, this depends upon the type of tissue involved and the degree of injury.

Abscess

An abscess is a localised collection of pus.

US

The appearance of an abscess on ultrasound is quite variable (**Figure 3.3**). It ranges from an anechoic to a hyperechoic lesion. There can be internal echoes, sediment, septae or gas. Its margin can range from round and generally well-defined to an irregular and lobulated lesion.

CT and MRI

The study is usually performed after contrast administration, if there are no contraindications. A mature well-encapsulated abscess on both CT and MRI will be seen as a ring-like enhancing lesion (**Figure 3.4**). MRI is better for delineating early changes – for example, in the stage of cerebritis before the formation of a cerebral abscess.

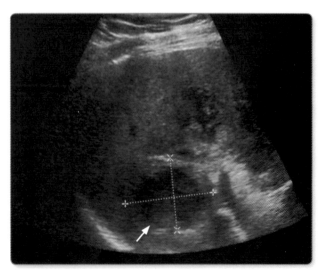

Figure 3.3 An abdominal ultrasound demonstrating a well-defined hypoechoic lesion containing internal echoes within the liver (arrow).

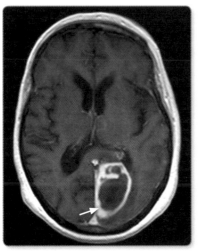

Figure 3.4 Axial CT scan post-contrast showing a ring enhancing brain abscess (arrow).

3.3 Effusion

An effusion is the seeping of serous, purulent or bloody fluid into a body cavity or tissue.

Pathophysiology

Effusions can be transudative or exudative:

- **Transudative effusions** are caused by systemic factors, such as left ventricular failure, liver or renal failure
- **Exudative effusion**, by contrast, is caused by alterations in local factors. Examples include malignant pleural effusion and middle ear effusion

Pleural effusion

A pleural effusion is fluid within the pleural cavity.

X-ray

A large free pleural effusion appears as a dependent opacity with lateral upward sloping of a meniscus-shaped contour (**Figure 3.5**). The diaphragmatic contour is partially or completely obliterated, depending on the amount of fluid. Small amounts of pleural fluid not readily seen on the standard frontal view may be demonstrated in a lateral decubitus view.

US

An effusion viewed on ultrasound can be totally anechoic, septated or echogenic, depending on the underlying cause. A transudative pleural effusion is usually anechoic (i.e. heart failure) (**Figure 3.6**). Infective/exudative pleural effusions can be septated, loculated and may contain debris. Within a haemorrhagic (i.e. echogenic) pleural effusion there may be increased internal echogenicity.

CT

Most CT examinations are performed with the patient supine, resulting in an accumulation of fluid posteriorly. Pleural effusions will be seen as crescent-shaped fluid-attenuating areas in the dependent portion of the hemithorax (**Figure 3.7**).

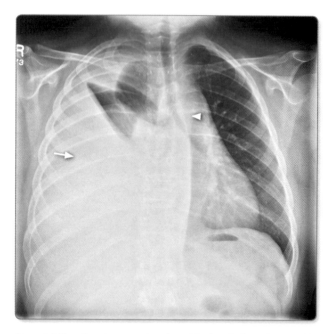

Figure 3.5 Chest X-ray demonstrating a large right pleural effusion (arrow) with mediastinal shift to the left (arrowhead).

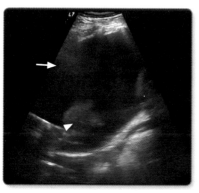

Figure 3.6 Ultrasound of the chest demonstrating a large pleural effusion (arrow) with collapse of the underlying lung (arrowhead).

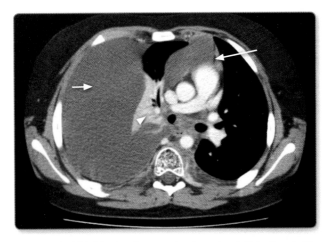

Figure 3.7 Axial CT of the chest demonstrating a large pleural effusion (arrow) with collapse of the underlying lung (arrowhead) and mediastinal shift to the left (long arrow).

MRI

The signal intensity of the pleural fluid depends on its biochemical characteristics (**Figure 3.8**). Non-haemorrhagic pleural effusions have low signal intensity on T1 images and high signal intensity on T2 images. It is possible to differentiate benign from malignant effusions on the basis of signal characteristics and contrast enhancement pattern.

3.4 Haemorrhage

Haemorrhage is defined as loss of blood from the circulatory system.

Pathophysiology

Haemorrhage can occur anywhere within the body, secondary to trauma. Haemorrhage can also be precipitated by trivial trauma if there are underlying factors that predispose the patient to bleeding (i.e. hypertension, bleeding diathesis, anticoagulants).

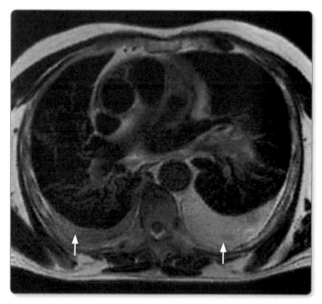

Figure 3.8 Axial MRI of the chest demonstrating bilateral pleural effusions with different signal intensities (arrows).

Intracranial haemorrhage as a result of a trivial head injury in a patient on warfarin is a good example.

CT

Acute haemorrhage appears hyperdense on CT due to the presence of macromolecule haemoglobin, which gives rise to a high electronic density (**Figure 3.9**). As haemoglobin is redistributed, the haemorrhage becomes isodense to adjacent tissue and hypodense thereafter.

MRI

It is difficult to demonstrate haemorrhage during the very acute stage on routine MRI sequences. Gradient echo sequence is very sensitive to blood products. Signal changes seen as a result of haemorrhage are dependent on the nature of the blood

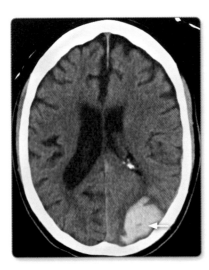

Figure 3.9 Axial CT of the brain, demonstrating a hyperdense area in the left occipital lobe, in keeping with acute haemorrhage (arrow).

product and the length of time since haemorrhage. Methaemoglobin seen in the early and late subacute stage is hyperintense or 'bright' on T1 and T2 images. Chronic haemorrhage is represented by haemosiderin and this has a characteristic low signal rim on both T1 and T2 images.

3.5 Thrombosis

A thrombus is a blood clot (a coagulation of fibrin, platelets and blood cells) formed in flowing blood.

Pathophysiology

Thrombosis can occur in an artery or vein. The factors contributing to the formation of a thrombus are changes in blood flow, blood viscosity and the integrity of the vessel wall.

Venous thrombosis results from the stagnation of blood within a vein. Many different risk factors predispose patients to venous thrombosis, including prolonged travel, trauma, hospitalisation, surgery and pregnancy. A part of the thrombus may dislodge (embolus) and travel via the blood vessels to other parts of the body. For example, an embolus from a deep vein thrombosis (DVT) can cause a pulmonary embolism.

US

The vein may be distended with echogenic material seen within the lumen in keeping with thrombus (**Figure 3.10a**). Two important features of thrombosis on ultrasound are loss

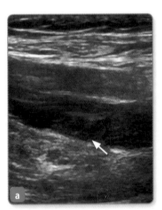

Figure 3.10 Thrombosis and thromboembolism. (a) Ultrasound of the common femoral vein demonstrating a distended vein with echogenic material in the lumen in keeping with thrombus (arrow). (b) Axial CT of the chest demonstrating a filling defect in the right pulmonary artery in keeping with pulmonary embolus (arrow).

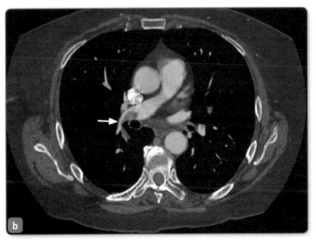

of compressibility and flow. This is well demonstrated on a duplex ultrasound of deep veins of the leg in a patient with DVT.

CT

Contrast enhancement is essential to demonstrate thromboembolism. It is seen as a filling defect with the normally contrast-filled vessel (**Figure 3.10b**).

MRI

Thrombosis results in the slow flow of blood and loss of the normal flow void within a vessel. Thrombosis is typically seen as a high signal within the vessel on T1 images.

3.6 Tumours and mass lesions

Pathophysiology

A tumour is a mass of tissue formed by abnormal growth and proliferation of cells in the body.

Malignant tumours are a class of diseases in which a group of cells display uncontrolled growth, invasion and sometimes metastasis. These three malignant properties of cancers differentiate them from benign tumours, which are self-limiting, and do not invade or metastasise.

US

Focal lesions distort normal anatomy (**Figure 3.11**). Ultrasound appearance can vary from echo-poor, echogenic to mixed echogenicity with necrosis.

CT and MRI

Neoplasms can be solitary, multifocal or diffusely infiltrative (**Figure 3.12**). Calcification, necrosis and contrast enhancement pattern help to characterise the lesion further. However, there are no set criteria that are capable of differentiating benign from malignant lesions. Hence, it is important to obtain tissue diagnosis, either by cytological or histological examination.

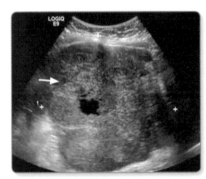

Figure 3.11 Ultrasound of pelvis demonstrating a large mass with mixed echogenicity (arrow).

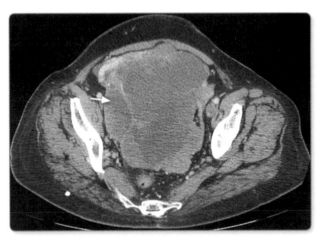

Figure 3.12 Axial CT of the pelvis demonstrating a large septated, cystic mass (arrow).

3.7 Calcifications

Calcification is the deposition of calcium salts in a tissue.

Pathophysiology

Calcification can be broadly classified as physiological and pathological:

- **Physiological calcification** occurs in the absence of any disease and is very common in brain structures like the pineal gland, choroid plexus and falx (**Figure 3.13**)
- **Pathological calcification** can be further classified as dystrophic or metastatic. Dystrophic calcification occurs locally in dying tissue despite normal serum levels of calcium and in the absence of derangements of calcium metabolism. In contrast, the deposition of calcium salts in otherwise normal tissue is known as metastatic calcification, and it almost always results from hypercalcaemia secondary to some disturbance of calcium metabolism

X-ray

Urinary tract calcification: the majority of urinary tract calcifications are radiopaque (**Figure 3.14a**). However, radiolucent calcifications will not be demonstrated on plain film and so other imaging modalities are employed. It is important to look for calcification in a patient with a history suggesting renal or ureteric colic.

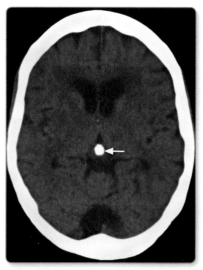

Figure 3.13 Axial CT of the brain demonstrating benign calcification in the pineal gland (arrow).

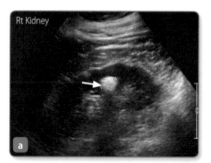

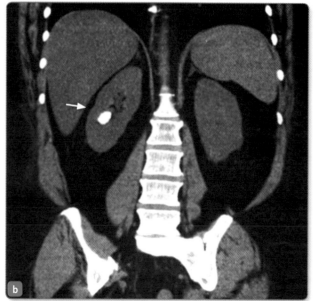

Figure 3.14 (a) Ultrasound of the right kidney demon-strating a renal calculus (arrow). (b) Coronal CT of the abdomen demonstrating right renal calculus (arrow).

US

Gallbladder calculi are not readily visible on plain radiographs and ultrasound is the modality of choice. Ultrasound may also be used to diagnose renal calculi and look for related complications i.e. hydronephrosis.

CT

Physiological calcification is best seen on CT examination of the head. The most common sites for physiological calcification include the pineal gland, choroid plexus, falx cerebri and tentorium.

Non-contrast CT of the renal tract is the method of choice to detect most types of renal calculi, including radiolucent calculus-like uric acid stones (**Figure 3.14b**).

3.8 Foreign bodies

Foreign bodies may be introduced in a range of ways, including inhalation, ingestion, through lacerations, as well as iatrogenic.

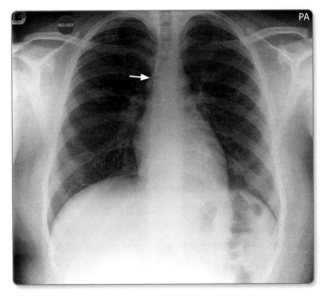

Figure 3.15 Chest X-ray demonstrating a linear foreign body at the carina (arrow), in keeping with an inhaled foreign body.

The imaging modality used to investigate the site of the foreign body and its related complications will depend on the clinical history, signs and symptoms.

X-ray

Radiopaque foreign bodies are readily seen on conventional radiographs (**Figure 3.15**). It is useful to obtain two perpendicular views (anteroposterior (AP) and lateral) on a radiograph to localise the exact location of the foreign body.

CT

CT is useful in demonstrating not only radiopaque but also many radiolucent foreign bodies. It also shows better the extent of soft tissue and visceral injury.

Gastrointestinal system

4.1 Key radiological anatomy

Solid abdominal viscera

Liver

Situated in the right upper quadrant, the liver Ⓐ is the largest organ in the body (**Figures 4.1–4.4**). Externally, the liver is divided into two anatomical lobes (right Ⓑ and left Ⓒ) by the attachment of the falciform ligament Ⓓ (**Figure 4.3**). Anatomically, the right lobe also comprises the quadrate and caudate lobes.

Functionally, the liver is divided into independent right and left lobes, each supplied by the right Ⓔ or left portal veins, right or left hepatic arteries, and each drained by the right or left hepatic ducts. The functional left lobe comprises the caudate lobe as well as a portion of the quadrate lobe. The lobes can be further subdivided into segments by the branches of the right and left hepatic arteries. Knowledge of segmental anatomy is important to localise pathology, aiding management.

Spleen

The spleen Ⓕ is situated in the left upper quadrant, relatively protected by the lower thoracic cage (**Figures 4.1–4.4**). The spleen is a very vascular organ supplied by the splenic artery (the largest branch of the coeliac axis) and is enclosed within a fibroelastic capsule (**Figure 4.3**).

Pancreas

The pancreas is divided into the head Ⓗ, uncinate process, neck Ⓘ, body Ⓙ and tail Ⓚ. The pancreas is a retroperitoneal structure, with the exception of the tail, which is related to the splenic hilum and lies in the splenorenal ligament. The normal pancreas is not normally visible on plain radiographs. As the

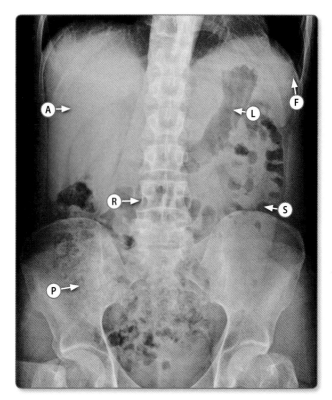

Figure 4.1 Abdominal radiograph demonstrates the liver (A), spleen (F), stomach (L), caecum (P), transverse colon (R) and descending colon (S).

pancreas lies transversely and obliquely, it is studied on sequential computed tomography (CT) images (**Figures 4.3** and **4.4**).

Hollow abdominal viscera

Oesophagus

The oesophagus is a muscular tube extending from the oropharynx to the stomach, approximately 25 cm in length. The gastro-oesophageal junction lies to the left of the T11 vertebral body.

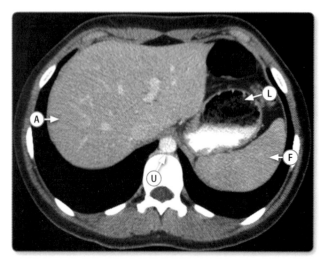

Figure 4.2 Axial abdominal CT scan demonstrates the liver Ⓐ, spleen Ⓕ, stomach Ⓛ and abdominal aorta Ⓤ.

Stomach and duodenum

The stomach Ⓘ is the dilated part of the digestive tract. It can hold 2–3 litres of ingested food and is divided into the cardia, fundus, body and pylorus. The pylorus controls gastric empty-ing into the first part (duodenal bulb) of the duodenum.

The duodenum Ⓜ is divided into four parts, all of which are retroperitoneal other than the duodenal bulb. The pancreatic duct and common bile duct empty into the second part of the duodenum. The fourth part of the duodenum joins the jejunum at the duodenojejunal junction, supported by the suspensory ligament of the duodenum (ligament of Treitz).

Gallbladder

The gallbladder Ⓝ (**Figure 4.4**) lies in the gallbladder fossa, an impression on the visceral surface of the liver. The cystic duct connects the gallbladder to the common hepatic duct to form the common bile duct.

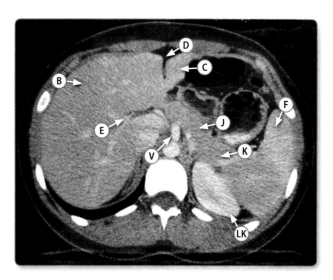

Figure 4.3 Axial abdominal CT scan demonstrates the right lobe of liver (B), left lobe of liver (C), falciform ligament (D), right portal vein (E) spleen (F), body of pancreas (J), tail of pancreas (K) and coeliac axis (V), left kidney (LK).

Small bowel

The small bowel (O) (**Figure 4.5**) comprises the jejunum and ileum, beginning at the duodenojejunal flexure, where the small intestine assumes a mesentery, and ending at the ileocaecal valve. The small bowel is centrally located, mobile and comprises circular mucosal folds (valvulae conniventes).

Large bowel

The large bowel (**Figures 4.5** and **4.6**) comprises the caecum (P), appendix (Q), ascending colon, transverse colon (R), descending colon (S) (**Figure 4.1**), sigmoid, rectum (T) (**Figure 4.6**) and anus. The large bowel is peripherally located, relatively fixed and of larger diameter in comparison to the small intestine. It is characterised by haustra, tenia coli and omental appendices. The transverse colon and sigmoid colon have a mesentery, hence are relatively mobile. The ascending and descending colons are retroperitoneal structures.

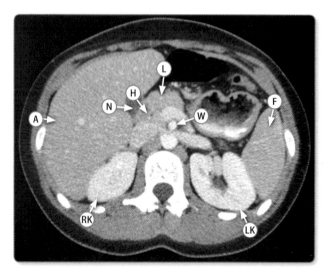

Figure 4.4 Axial abdominal CT scan demonstrates the liver Ⓐ, spleen Ⓕ, head of pancreas Ⓗ, neck of pancreas Ⓛ, gallbladder Ⓝ and superior mesenteric artery Ⓦ, right kidney ⓇⓀ, left kidney ⓁⓀ.

Vascular structure

The abdominal aorta Ⓤ begins at the aortic hiatus, an opening posterior to the diaphragm at the level of T12. The abdominal aorta descends to the left of the vertebral bodies to the level of L4 where it bifurcates into the common iliac arteries. The abdominal aorta gives rise to visceral and parietal arteries. Major unpaired visceral branches (**Figures 4.2–4.5**) are the coeliac axis Ⓥ, superior mesenteric artery (SMA) Ⓦ, and inferior mesenteric artery (IMA) Ⓧ. Paired visceral branches are the suprarenal, renal and gonadal arteries. The parietal branches supply the posterior abdominal wall and diaphragm.

4.2 Trauma

Abdominal trauma is a common presentation within the emergency department, with injuries resulting from both blunt and penetrating injuries.

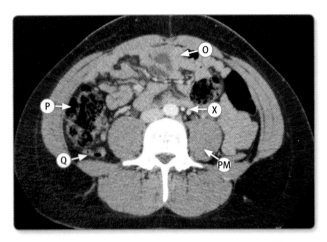

Figure 4.5 Axial abdominal CT scan demonstrates small bowel loops (O), caecum (P), appendix (Q) and inferior mesenteric artery (X), psoas muscle (PM).

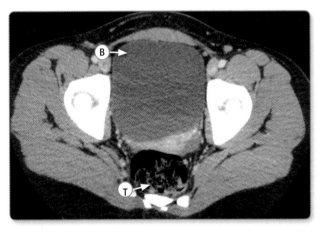

Figure 4.6 Axial abdominal CT scan demonstrates the rectum (T) and bladder (B).

Blunt abdominal trauma

Blunt abdominal trauma is usually the result of road traffic collisions, falls and crush injuries. The spleen is the most commonly injured intra-abdominal organ, followed by the liver. Depending on the severity of injury, patients with a history of trauma can present with abdominal pain, bruising and hypotension secondary to blood loss.

Key facts

Splenic injury This is associated with injuries to other solid abdominal viscera. Underlying splenic injury should be suspected in patients with left-sided rib fractures or left renal injury. Minor trauma can lead to splenic rupture if there is underlying pathology that has resulted in splenomegaly.

Splenic injuries are graded in severity based on the extent of the subcapsular haematoma and depth of laceration. Severe injuries involve a completely shattered spleen with devascularisation due to disruption of the hilar vessels.

Liver The liver is the second most frequently injured organ in blunt abdominal trauma, with the right lobe more susceptible to injury than the left. The severity of liver injury depends upon the extent of subcapsular haematoma, depth of liver laceration and the number of liver segments or degree of lobe injured.

Road traffic accidents Blunt abdominal trauma is common in children involved in road traffic collisions due to seat belt injuries or bicycle handlebar injuries. This type of trauma results in injury to the jejunum distal to the ligament of Treitz and duodenum. Clinical findings include tender abdomen, bruising, tachycardia, increased temperature and reduced urine output.

Radiographic findings

US Ultrasound (US) of the liver or spleen may demonstrate a localised area of increased intraparenchymal

Clinical insight

Patients may undergo focused assessment with sonography for trauma (FAST) to assess for free fluid, an indicator of underlying injury. A common site for free fluid to collect is in the subhepatic space.

echogenicity in keeping with acute haematoma. There can also be heterogenous echogenicity of the liver/spleen in keeping with a vascular injury. This can be associated with free fluid within the abdomen.

CT CT will demonstrate a hypoattenuating haematoma and laceration, subcapsular haematoma and haemoperitoneum. There can be active extravasation of contrast medium in keeping with active haemorrhage best seen on arterial phase scans.

Hypovolaemia can result in 'hypoperfusion complex'. Intense vasoconstriction results in a small aorta and mesenteric arteries. A decrease in venous return results in a flattened inferior vena cava. There will be marked enhancement of the pancreas and adrenal glands.

Key signs

- Irregular hypodense lacerations (**Figure 4.7**)
- Subcapsular haematoma (**Figure 4.7** and **4.8**)
- Active extravasation of contrast in keeping with active haemorrhage (**Figure 4.8**)
- Associated injuries to other organs
- Hypoperfusion complex

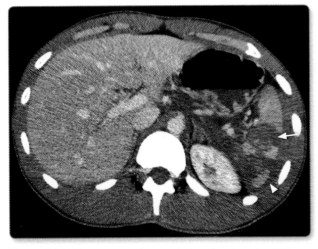

Figure 4.7 Axial CT post-contrast demonstrates hypodense, irregular splenic lacerations (arrow) with subcapsular haematoma (arrowhead).

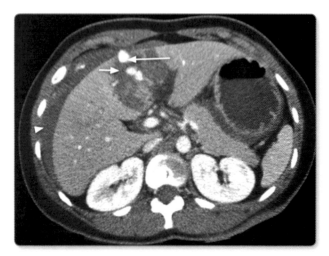

Figure 4.8 Axial CT post-contrast demonstrates hypodense liver laceration (arrow), subcapsular haematoma (arrowhead) and active extravasation of contrast in keeping with active haemorrhage (long arrow).

Management

Further management of the patient will depend on the severity of the injury sustained and its location. If active haemorrhage has been demonstrated, then there may be a role for interventional vascular radiology and embolectomy.

Penetrating abdominal trauma

Penetrating abdominal trauma can lead to significant injury of organs, bowel and vasculature, in the path of the projectile or stab wound.

Key facts

- The site of injury is important as posterior wounds are more likely to cause retroperitoneal injury. Thoracoabdominal injuries should be evaluated carefully for an injury to the diaphragm

- Haemodynamically unstable patients may need to go straight to theatre. There should not be a delay to urgent intervention in order to perform imaging

Radiographic findings

US A FAST scan may have been performed by the trauma team to look for free fluid. However, US does not have a role in penetrating trauma due to decreased specificity and sensitivity for detecting injury.

CT This will demonstrate the entry and, if present, exit wounds, the missile path and the extent of injury. Foreign bodies/projectiles can be seen if still lodged in the abdomen. Bowel injury may result in pneumoperitoneum, although subtle injury to the bowel may not be detected by CT, and a high index of suspicion is required. Injuries to organs will result in subcapsular haematoma, lacerations and active haemorrhage. Patients can be in hypovolaemic shock, displaying signs of hypoperfusion complex.

Key signs
- Entry +/– exit wounds (**Figure 4.9a**)
- Haemoperitoneum and pneumoperitoneum
- Hypodense parenchymal injury/laceration (**Figure 4.9b**)
- Subcapsular haematoma
- Active haemorrhage
- Hypoperfusion complex

Management
Urgent surgery is indicated in unstable patients. Surgery should not be delayed in order to perform imaging.

4.3 Acute inflammation

A very common clinical presentation encountered is acute abdominal pain. Patients present with a range of symptoms and signs, providing diagnostic clues to the underlying inflammatory process.

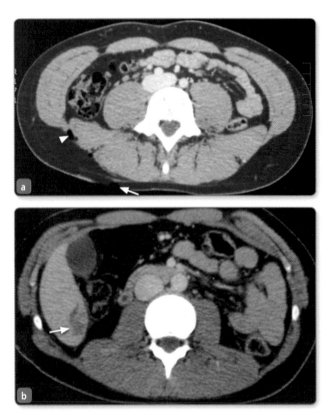

Figure 4.9 (a) Axial CT post-contrast demonstrates the site of penetrating trauma (stab wound) (arrow) and air within the subcutaneous tissues demarcating the path of the stab wound (arrowhead) (b) Axial CT post-contrast demonstrates a hypodense, irregular liver laceration as a result of the penetrating trauma (arrow).

Gallstones and related complications

Gallstones are a common cause of acute right upper abdominal pain, with acute cholecystitis a common reason for hospital admission. There are many different factors associated with developing gallstones, including diet, age, gender, geography and alcohol intake. The majority of gallstones are composed of cholesterol (approximately 80%).

Key facts

Acute cholecystitis usually results from gallstone impaction in the gallbladder neck or cystic duct. Complications of acute cholecystitis include emphysematous cholecystitis due to gas-forming organisms. Perforation of the gallbladder wall results in pericholecystic abscess, a fluid collection near the fundus of the gallbladder

Further complications of gallstones include acute pancreatitis, gallstone ileus and Mirizzi syndrome, in which a stone impacted in the cystic duct causes narrowing of the common bile duct and subsequent biliary obstruction

Ascending cholangitis results from obstruction of the biliary tree, superimposed by a bacterial infection. The patient can present with Charcot's triad of right upper quadrant pain, fever and obstructive jaundice

Radiographic findings

Plain radiograph Approximately 10–15% of gallstones are radio-opaque and can be seen on plain radiographs. Gallstone ileus may be demonstrated on plain radiograph with the 'Rigler triad'. This comprises of small bowel obstruction, air within the biliary tree and a large gallstone located in an ectopic position.

US Ultrasound is the modality of choice for diagnosing gallstones and their related complications. Gallstones produce a highly reflective echo from their anterior surface, and demonstrate mobility and posterior acoustic shadowing (**Figure 4.10**). Acute cholecystitis results in gallbladder wall thickening (>3 mm) and pericholecystic fluid, with a positive sonographic Murphy's sign.

CT/ MRI CT is useful for imaging complications, including gallbladder perforation (**Figure 4.11**), empyema and gallstone ileus (**Figure 4.12**). Magnetic resonance imaging (MRI) is useful for determining if there is an obstructing common bile duct calculus, prior to endoscopic retrograde cholangiopancreatography (ERCP).

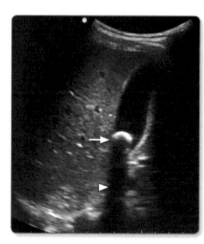

Figure 4.10 Ultrasound of the gallbladder demonstrates a highly reflective echo from there anterior surface of a solitary gallstone (arrow) and posterior acoustic shadowing (arrowhead).

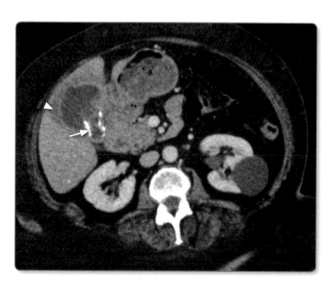

Figure 4.11 Axial CT post-contrast demonstrates a gallstone in the neck of the gallbladder (arrow). The gallbladder wall is irregular with surrounding hypodensity due to perforation (arrowhead).

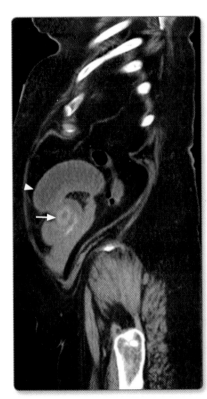

Figure 4.12 Sagittal CT post-contrast demonstrates a large gallstone (arrow) within the small bowel, resulting in small bowel obstruction (arrowhead).

Key signs

- Echogenic, mobile and shadowing calculi
- Sonographic Murphy's sign
- Gallbladder wall thickening, pericholecystic fluid and gall-bladder perforation
- Dilated intrahepatic bile ducts and common bile duct
- Rigler triad – incomplete/complete small bowel obstruction, biliary tree air (**Figure 4.13**) and ectopic calcified gallstone

Management

Management will depend on the patient's presentation and related complications.

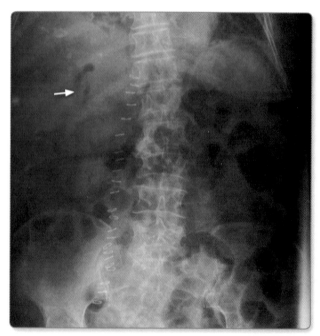

Figure 4.13 Abdominal radiograph demonstrates the air within the biliary tree (arrow), which was as a result of recent surgery.

Acute pancreatitis

Acute pancreatitis is inflammation of the pancreas. Activated pancreatic enzymes leak from the ductal system, resulting in pancreatic autodigestion and lysis of adjacent structures. Patients usually present with epigastric pain that radiates to the back, nausea and vomiting, and abdominal distension.

Key facts

- Gallstones are the commonest cause of acute pancreatitis, followed by alcohol and iatrogenic causes (post-ERCP)
- Complications of acute pancreatitis include haemorrhagic pancreatitis, pseudocyst or abscess formation, and pseudoaneurysm

Radiographic findings

US Ultrasound is useful for determining the underlying cause for acute pancreatitis, i.e. gallstones. However, localised ileus due to surrounding inflammation may make ultrasound very difficult to perform.

CT CT is recommended for cases where the diagnosis is in doubt, severe clinical pancreatitis and patients that are failing to improve on conservative medical management. CT will demonstrate focal or diffuse pancreatic oedema with poor definition of the gland. There will be surrounding peripancreatic inflammation and free fluid, the extent of which depends on the severity of pancreatitis. Contrast scan will demonstrate any areas of pancreatic necrosis, which will not enhance (**Figure 4.14**). In severe necrotising pancreatitis there will be gland necrosis with free gas (**Figure 4.15**).

Key signs
- Pancreatic oedema, peripancreatic inflammation and free fluid

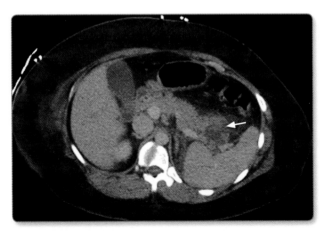

Figure 4.14 Axial CT post-contrast demonstrates oedema and irregularity of the tail of pancreas. There is decreased enhancement of the tail in keeping with acute pancreatitis (arrow).

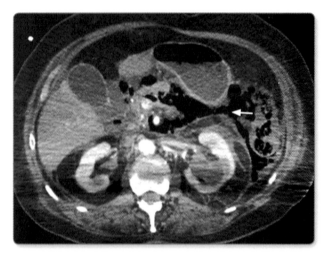

Figure 4.15 Axial CT post-contrast demonstrates extensive gas surrounding the pancreas due to acute necrotising pancreatitis (arrow).

- Ill-defined gland
- Fluid collections (**Figure 4.16**)
- Necrosis
- Pseudoaneurysm formation

Management

Acute pancreatitis is managed conservatively. However, if intra-abdominal collections form there may be a role for radiological drainage.

Acute appendicitis

Acute appendicitis is a common acute surgical presentation. The appendiceal lumen may become obstructed by lymphoid hyperplasia, faecoliths, foreign bodies and less common strictures and malignancy.

Clinical insight

Clinical diagnosis of acute appendicitis can be difficult in the elderly, very young and females, especially as patients may present with non-specific symptoms. A high index of clinical suspicion is required as a delayed diagnosis can lead to an increased perforation rate.

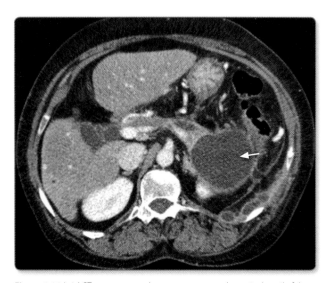

Figure 4.16 Axial CT post-contrast demonstrates a pseudocyst in the tail of the pancreas (arrow).

Key facts

Patients usually present with acute abdominal pain, nausea and vomiting, low-grade fever and diarrhoea. Initially, there is poorly localised visceral epigastric/periumbilical abdominal pain, which then migrates into the right lower quadrant over the appendix (McBurney's point).

Radiographic findings

Plain radiograph Acute appendicitis is not an indication for plain radiograph as findings can be very non-specific. There may be a laminated calcified appendicolith in the right lower quadrant, which in patients presenting with abdominal pain presents a very high probability of appendicitis. Sentinel loops of bowel may be present in the right lower quadrant, due to localised inflammatory change leading to paralytic ileus.

US Ultrasound is useful to help confirm acute appendicitis or to diagnose other causes of right iliac fossa pain, especially in female patients who may be presenting with gynaecological pathology.

Graded compression ultrasound is the modality of choice to visualise a non-compressible, inflamed appendix, a blind-ending tubular structure (**Figure 4.17a** and **b**). Using the ultrasound probe to apply graded compression will displace overlying bowel loops and aid examination of the appendix. An appendix diameter of more than 6 mm is very specific for appendicitis. There may be a distended lumen with an appendicolith seen as a hyperechoic focus with posterior acoustic shadowing. Surrounding inflammatory change will be seen as increased echogenicity within the pericaecal fat as well as free fluid.

CT CT may be useful if the appendix has not been visualised on ultrasound or if the findings are equivocal. CT will demonstrate a distended appendix with a thickened wall, appendicolith and surrounding inflammatory change (**Figure 4.17c**).

Key signs
- Non-compressible, blind-ending tubular structure
- > 6 mm in diameter
- Appendicolith
- Surrounding inflammatory change

Management
Patients should be referred to the surgical team for appendicectomy.

4.4 Bowel obstruction

Bowel dilatation can result from a mechanical intestinal obstruction or a paralytic ileus. Differentiating between small bowel obstruction and large bowel obstruction is important as it aids further management (**Table 4.1**).

Small bowel obstruction
Mechanical small bowel obstruction is due to adhesions from previous surgery in the majority of cases, followed by hernia.

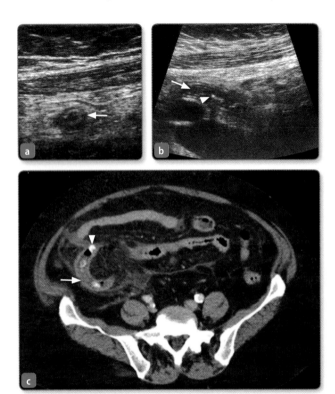

Figure 4.17 (a) Transverse ultrasound demonstrates a thickened appendix. (b) Longitudinal ultrasound demonstrates a distended appendix (arrow) containing faecoliths (arrowhead) (c) Axial CT post-contrast demonstrates a thick walled, distended appendix (arrow) containing appendicoliths (arrowhead). There is surrounding inflammatory change due to acute appendicitis.

Other causes include gallstone ileus, closed loop obstruction, masses and intussusception.

Key facts

- Small bowel obstruction can lead to devastating complications of perforation, ischaemia and infarction, with significant morbidity and mortality

Small Bowel	Large Bowel
Calibre 3 – 5cm	Calibre > 5 cm
Central loops	Peripheral loops
Valvulae conniventes	Haustra
Multiple loops	Fewer loops

Table 4.1 Differences between the small and large bowel that can help distinguish them on imaging.

- Symptoms and signs at presentation include generalised acute abdominal pain, nausea and vomiting, abdominal distension and 'tinkling' bowel sounds
- Early surgical input and imaging are important in diagnosis and management

Radiographic findings

Plain radiograph Supine abdominal radiographs will demonstrate dilated central gas-filled small bowel loops (**Figure 4.18**). Erect abdominal radiographs may demonstrate multiple fluid levels within the dilated small bowel. There may be a clue to the underlying cause, for example, the presence of a hernia (**Figure 4.19**).

If the bowel obstruction has been complicated by perforation, then signs of pneumoperitoneum may be present. On erect chest radiograph, free gas under the diaphragm is a common finding (**Figure 4.20**). On supine radiograph, free gas may be seen outlining both sides of the bowel wall (Rigler's sign) (**Figure 4.21**). The falciform ligament sign demonstrates free gas outlining the falciform ligament. The football sign is seen more commonly in neonates with free gas outlining the peritoneal cavity.

CT CT will demonstrate dilated small bowel loops (**Figure 4.22**), as well as the underlying cause for the small bowel obstruction, including hernias (**Figure 4.23**), gallstones and masses. In cases of adhesions there will be an abrupt change in the calibre of the small bowel loop. Pneumoperitoneum will be demonstrated as free gas.

Key signs

- Dilated small bowel loops
- Abrupt calibre change at level of obstruction
- Free gas under the diaphragm on erect chest radiograph
- Signs of pneumoperitoneum

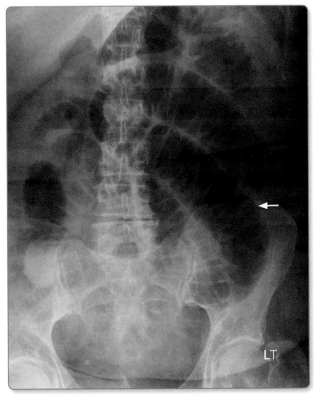

Figure 4.18 Abdominal radiograph demonstrates small bowel obstruction (arrow).

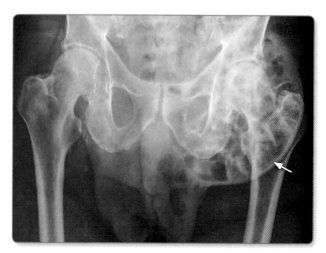

Figure 4.19 Pelvic radiograph demonstrates a large left inguinal hernia containing bowel loops (arrow).

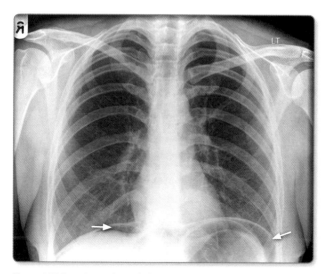

Figure 4.20 Erect chest radiograph demonstrates pneumoperitoneum as free gas beneath the diaphragms (arrows).

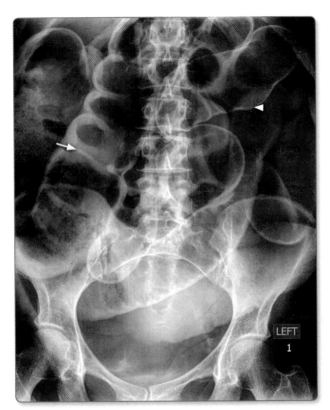

Figure 4.21 Abdominal radiograph demonstrates small bowel obstruction (arrow) with Rigler's sign of pneumoperitoneum (arrowhead).

Management

Urgent surgery is indicated if a strangulated hernia is the cause of a small bowel obstruction or if complications are present. In other cases conservative management may be appropriate.

Large bowel obstruction

Large bowel obstruction commonly results from colonic masses, followed by diverticulitis and volvulus.

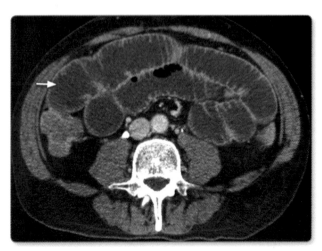

Figure 4.22 Axial CT post-contrast demonstrates a small bowel obstruction with distended, fluid filled small bowel loops (arrow).

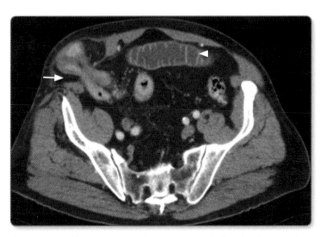

Figure 4.23 Axial CT post-contrast demonstrates a right Spigelian hernia, with the hernial sac containing a small bowel loop (arrow). There is associated small bowel obstruction as a result (arrowhead).

Key facts

- Colorectal cancer is the most common cancer of the gastro-intestinal (GI) tract and should be considered in all patients presenting with large bowel obstruction
- Volvulus of the colon occurs in parts that are relatively mobile, with the sigmoid and caecum mostly affected

Radiographic findings

Plain radiograph Abdominal radiographs will demonstrate dilated, peripheral, gas-filled large bowel with haustra. Signs of pneumoperitoneum may be present if perforation has occurred.

Caecal volvulus results in a distended gas- and fluid-filled caecal pole lying in the left upper quadrant (**Figure 4.24**). The small bowel may be distended and gas-filled. Sigmoid volvulus results in a grossly distended loop of bowel, extending to the diaphragm (**Figure 4.25**).

> **Clinical insight**
>
> In patients with known colitis, toxic megacolon should be considered, as perforation and peritonitis are common complications. On plain abdominal radiograph, a dilated colon of >5.5 cm (usually the transverse colon) with mucosal islands is seen.

CT CT will demonstrate the dilated loops of large bowel as well as demonstrating the underlying cause. In caecal and sigmoid volvulus there will be a classic 'swirl' in the mesentery at the site of the torsion (**Figure 4.26**). Complications of large bowel obstruction, which include perforation, ischaemia and infarction, may be demonstrated.

Key signs

- Dilated large bowel >5 cm calibre
- Mass
- Caecal or sigmoid volvulus (**Figure 4.27**)
- Toxic megacolon
- Pneumoperitoneum (**Figure 4.28**)

Management

Surgical referral is required, with further management depending on the cause of the large bowel obstruction. There may

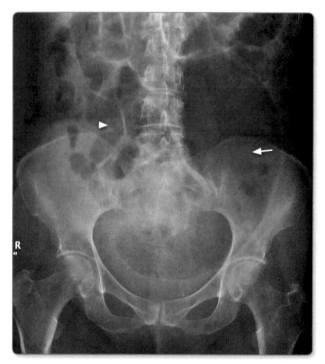

Figure 4.24 Abdominal radiograph demonstrates caecal volvulus. The caecum now lies on the left side of the abdomen (arrow) with associated distension of the small bowel loops (arrowhead).

be a need for decompression or defunctioning. In the case of uncomplicated sigmoid volvulus a flatus tube may be used for decompression.

4.5 Acute mesenteric ischaemia

Acute mesenteric ischaemia is caused by insufficient blood flow to the intestine. Causes include arterial occlusion, venous occlusion and bowel obstruction. Patients present with initially crampy, then continuous, abdominal pain, vomiting

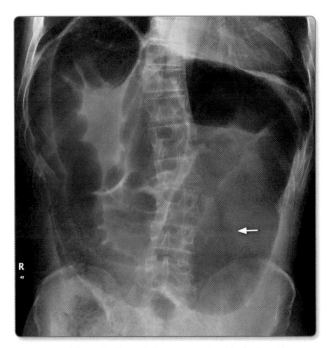

Figure 4.25 Abdominal radiograph demonstrates sigmoid volvulus, with a grossly distended sigmoid colon extending to the diaphragm (arrow).

and bloody diarrhoea. There may be an underlying history of cardiac disease (e.g. atrial fibrillation) predisposing to embolisation.

Key facts
- The splenic flexure and proximal descending colon are most commonly affected
- Irreversible bowel ischaemia will result in transmural infarction, bowel perforation and is associated with a high mortality rate

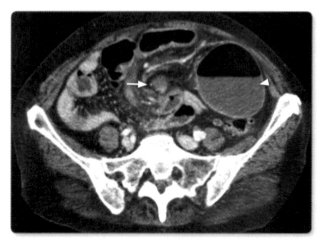

Figure 4.26 Axial CT post-contrast demonstrates the classic 'swirl' appearance of the mesentry in caecal volvulus (arrow). The caecal pole is lying on the left of the abdomen (arrowhead).

Radiographic findings

Plain radiograph Plain abdominal radiographs demonstrate dilated bowel loops and bowel wall thickening (thumbprinting). A sign of irreversible ischaemia is pneumatosis coli, as luminal gas dissects through compromised mucosa into the bowel wall. There may be propagation of intramural gas into the mesenteric vein and portal vein, demonstrated as linear branching lucencies overlying the liver (**Figure 4.29**). Pneumoperitoneum will be present if there has been perforation of the infarcted bowel.

CT CT will demonstrate poorly enhancing, dilated bowel loops (**Figure 4.30**) with circumferential bowel wall thickening in the affected territory. There may be engorgement of the mesenteric vessels and ascites due to venous congestion. Intramural gas, portal venous gas and pneumoperitoneum may be present in very severe cases (**Figure 4.31**). There may be thrombus/embolus within the mesenteric vessels, indicating the underlying cause for the mesenteric ischaemia.

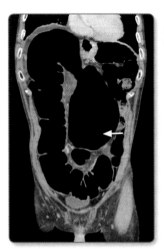

Figure 4.27 Coronal CT post-contrast demonstrates a sigmoid volvulus (arrow).

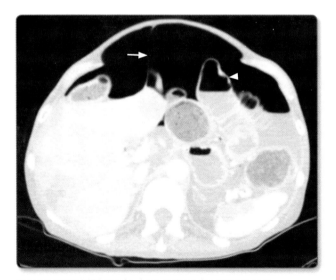

Figure 4.28 Axial CT (viewed on lung windows) demonstrates gross pneumoperitoneum. The free gas outlines the falciform ligament (arrow) and the bowel (arrowhead) as seen on plain radiograph as the falciform ligament sign and Riglers sign.

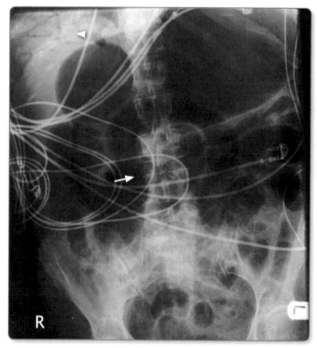

Figure 4.29 Abdominal radiograph demonstrates dilated central small bowel loops in keeping with bowel obstruction. There are branching linear lucencies overlying the liver shadow in keeping with portal venous gas (arrowhead).

Key signs
- Dilated bowel loops
- Thumbprinting/thickening of bowel loops
- Poorly enhancing bowel loops
- Pneumatosis coli, portal venous gas and pneumoperitoneum

Management
Early diagnosis and management are crucial to try to prevent bowel infarction.

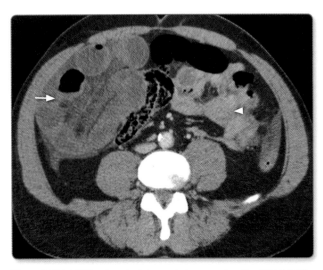

Figure 4.30 Axial CT post-contrast demonstrates non-enhancing, dilated small bowel loops with surrounding free fluid (arrow). The appearances are of infarcted bowel, compared to normal bowel on left side (arrowhead).

4.6 Acute gastrointestinal haemorrhage

Acute GI haemorrhage is a medical/surgical emergency needing prompt evaluation and treatment. Depending on the site and extent of haemorrhage, patients can present with haematemesis, malaena, haematochezia, tachycardia, hypotension and syncope.

Key facts

- Upper GI haemorrhage is bleeding proximal to the ligament of Treitz. Causes of upper GI haemorrhage include oesophageal varices and peptic ulcer disease. Patients with upper GI haemorrhage should initially be investigated by oesophageal gastro endoscopy (OGD)
- Lower GI haemorrhage is bleeding distal to the ligament of Treitz. Colorectal haemorrhage is most common secondary to diverticula and angiodysplasia and patients may be investigated with colonoscopy

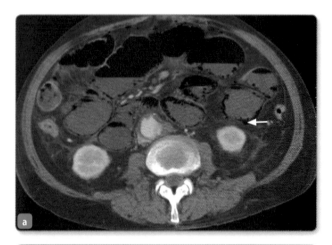

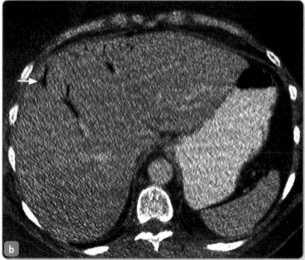

Figure 4.31 (a) Axial CT post-contrast demonstrates dilated small bowel loops with intramural gas (arrow). (b) Axial CT post-contrast demonstrates portal venous gas as linear branching, air attenuation within the periphery of the liver (arrow).

- Conventional angiography and CT angiography are useful for identifying the site of bleeding

Radiographic findings

CT angiography and conventional angiography CT angiography performed during active haemorrhage is useful to identify the site of bleeding and to plan intervention. A non contrast scan allows differentiation from other causes of high attenuation within the bowel i.e. calcification, when compared to the arterial scan (**Figure 4.32a**). On arterial phase imaging, the site

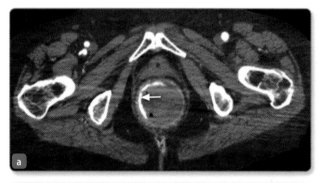

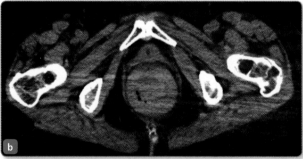

Figure 4.32 (a) Axial CT post-contrast demonstrates high attenuation within the lumen of the rectum, in keeping with active haemorrhage (arrow), which was not present on the non-contrast scan (b).

of active haemorrhage will be seen as high attenuation within the bowel wall/lumen **(Figure 4.32b)**.

Key signs
- High attenuation within the bowel lumen on CT
- Extravasation of contrast media on conventional angiography

Management
Mesenteric angiography +/− embolisation may be indicated if the patient is actively bleeding.

Genitourinary system

5.1 Key radiological anatomy

Urinary tract

Kidneys

The kidneys (right Ⓐ, left Ⓑ) are retroperitoneal structures, lying obliquely in the paravertebral gutters. Each kidney normally measures 10–15 cm in length. On plain radiograph, perirenal fat makes the outline of the kidneys visible (**Figure 5.1**). Ultrasound (US) of the kidneys demonstrates the cortex Ⓒ, renal sinus Ⓓ and hilum Ⓔ (**Figure 5.2**).

Ureters

Each ureter is 25–30 cm in length from renal pelvis to the bladder. The abdominal ureter lies anterior to the medial edge of the psoas muscle Ⓕ (**Figure 5.1**). The ureter enters the pelvis at the bifurcation of the common iliac arteries, anterior to the sacroiliac joints, and enters the bladder posterolaterally.

Bladder

The urinary bladder Ⓖ is a muscular hollow viscus. It is located superior and posterior to the pubic bones and is an extraperitoneal structure. Imaging modalities used to assess the bladder include US, computed tomography (CT), magnetic resonance imaging (MRI) and fluoroscopy (**Figure 5.3**).

Testis

The testes are paired oval glands located within the scrotal sac, suspended by the spermatic cord. The testes Ⓗ are covered by a fibrous capsule, the tunica albuginae. The epididymis Ⓘ is a convoluted duct on the posterior surface of the testis, responsible for concentrating, storing and transporting sperm.

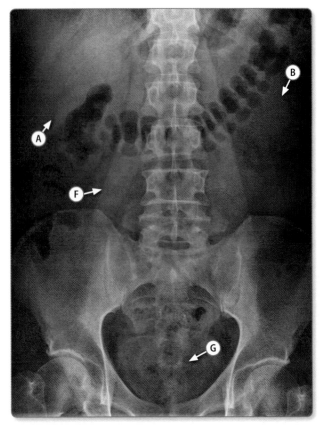

Figure 5.1 Abdominal radiograph demonstrates the outlines of the right kidney (A), left kidney (B), psoas muscle (F) and bladder (G).

Both testis and epididymis are covered by the tunica vaginalis (**Figure 5.4**).

Ovaries

The ovaries (J) are paired oval organs that lie in close contact with the infundibulum of the fallopian tube, on the posterior

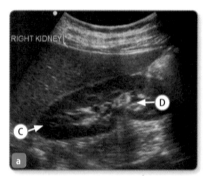

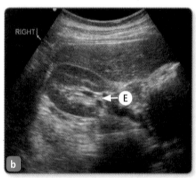

Figure 5.2 (a) Longitudinal ultrasound scan of the right kidney demonstrates the renal cortex (C) and renal sinus (D). (b) Transverse ultrasound scan of the right kidney demonstrates the renal hilum (E).

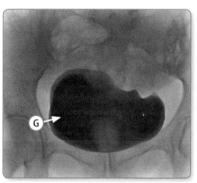

Figure 5.3 Fluoroscopy of the urinary bladder. There is a catheter in situ and contrast has filled the bladder (G).

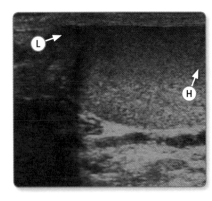

Figure 5.4 Ultrasound scan of the scrotum demonstrates a testis (H) and epididymus (L).

surface of the broad ligament. Each ovary is attached to the broad ligament by a mesovarium and the uterus by the ovarian ligament. The normal ovary will demonstrate multiple peripheral follicles (**Figure 5.5**).

5.2 Renal trauma

Renal injury occurs in approximately 10% of blunt and penetrating trauma. A high index of suspicion for renal injury is needed in patients presenting with back and flank trauma. Patients may be haemodynamically unstable, presenting with haematuria.

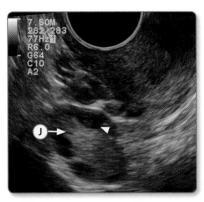

Figure 5.5 Ultrasound scan of the pelvis demonstrates an ovary (J) with follicles (arrowhead).

Key facts

- Blunt trauma to the kidney commonly results from a direct blow, with the kidney injured by the lower ribs
- Renal injury is very often associated with other organ injury
- Injury to the ureter commonly occurs at the pelviureteric junction, due to overstretching in hyperflexion or compression against the vertebral transverse processes

Radiographic findings

US Renal ultrasound can be used to identify and assess renal injury, however is not very sensitive and should not be used routinely.

CT CT is the modality of choice to assess renal parenchymal injury, vasculature, perinephric haematoma (**Figure 5.6**) and active haemorrhage. Renal injury can be graded, with the severest injury resulting in fragmentation of the kidney, devascularisation, large perinephric haematoma, active

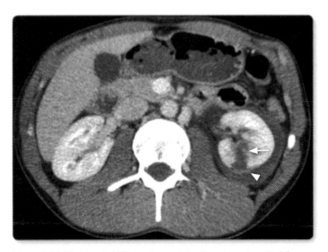

Figure 5.6 Axial abdominal CT scan demonstrates hypodense, irregular left kidney laceration (arrow) with subcapsular haematoma (arrowhead).

haemorrhage and extravasation of urine. A delayed scan (CT urogram) will show contrast within the collecting system and ureter, demonstrating urine leak, if present.

Key signs
- Hypodense parenchymal injury
- Perinephric haematoma
- Active haemorrhage
- Active extravasation of urine

Management
Patients with severe renal injury will need urgent radiological or surgical intervention. Minor degrees of renal injury can be treated conservatively.

5.3 Bladder trauma

The majority of bladder injuries are associated with pelvic fractures (70%), with the severity of pelvic injury correlating with the possibility of bladder injury. Patients with significant bladder injuries will have frank haematuria. Bladder injuries can range from contusions (most common) to bladder rupture.

Key facts
Contusion to the bladder results in an intramural haematoma, with decreased distension of the bladder. The intramural haematoma will be demonstrated as a crescentic filling defect in a contrast-filled bladder.

Extraperitoneal bladder rupture is the most common type of rupture, followed by intraperitoneal bladder rupture. Extraperitoneal bladder rupture occurs close to the bladder base, whereas intraperitoneal bladder rupture usually occurs at the dome of the bladder.

Clinical insight

Patients with pelvic fractures may have significant internal haemorrhage due to injury to pelvic vessels. The main priority in managing these patients is to control the active haemorrhage. Following this, urethral injury should be investigated and, when safe to do so, bladder injury.

Radiographic findings

Conventional cystography This should only be performed once urethral injury has been excluded and it is safe to proceed with retrograde bladder catheterisation.

CT cystogram On delayed phase scanning, the bladder will fill with contrast medium. This may demonstrate contusions as a focal thickening of the bladder wall. Extravasation of contrast will be in keeping with bladder rupture. CT is also helpful to assess other associated injuries and the extent of pelvic injury. Limitations of this technique include inadequate bladder distension by the contrast and hence bladder injury cannot be confirmed or excluded reliably.

Key signs
- Focal bladder wall thickening
- Contrast extravasation from bladder
- Pelvic fractures and associated haemorrhage (**Figures 5.7**)
- Indeterminate scan due to inadequate bladder distension

Management
Urological assessment is required for patients where bladder injuries are suspected.

5.4 Urinary tract calculi

A large majority of patients presenting with acute loin pain will have renal tract calculi. Patients will present with severe loin pain (which may radiate to the groin) and microscopic haematuria.

Key facts
- The majority of urinary tract calculi are radio-opaque on plain radiograph. Calculi formed from urate or xanthines are radiolucent (3–4%)
- Staghorn calculi are formed commonly by struvite, in the presence of infection and alkaline urine
- Complications of urinary tract calculi include obstruction, ureteral stricture, renal infection and decreased renal function

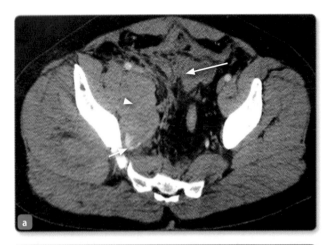

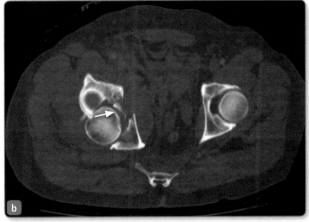

Figure 5.7 (a) Axial CT post contrast demonstrates a pelvic fracture resulting in active haemorrhage (short arrow) and associated pelvic haematoma (arrowhead). There is increased stranding around the urinary bladder, suspicious of bladder injury (long arrow). (b) Axial CT (bone windows) demonstrates the pelvic fracture involving the right acetabulum (arrow).

Radiographic findings

Plain radiograph Calculi may be seen on plain radiograph (**Figure 5.8**) as radio opacities overlying the renal shadows or the psoas shadow, along the tips of the transverse processes of the lumbar vertebrae. However, there may be difficulties in accurate detection. Reasons for this include: smaller calculi, overlying bowel gas and differentiation from other calcifications.

US Ultrasound not only helps detect renal calculi, but also allows assessment for possible complications (i.e. obstruction/hydrone-

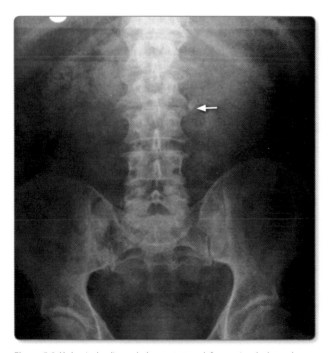

Figure 5.8 Abdominal radiograph demonstrates a left ureteric calculus at the level of the L2/L3 intervertebral disc (arrow).

phrosis and infection) (**Figure 5.9**). Ultrasound will demonstrate a hyperechoic calculus with posterior acoustic shadowing. The use of colour Doppler on the calculus will demonstrate a 'twinkling' artefact, which may help to confirm the presence of calculi.

CT Patients are more commonly investigated for urinary tract calculi with non-contrast CT. CT will demonstrate high attenuation calculi within the urinary tract. Ureteric calculi can be accurately localised and may be surrounded by soft tissue forming a halo (rim sign). Findings of obstruction of the kidney can also be assessed. This includes dilatation of the pelvicaliceal system and ureter proximal to the calculus and perinephric soft tissue stranding due to oedema of the perinephric fat (**Figure 5.10**). A negative CT for calculi, will also allow assessment for other potential causes of pain.

Key signs
- Radio-opaque calculi on radiograph
- Hyperechoic calculi on ultrasound
- High attenuation calculi on CT (**Figures 5.10** and **5.11**)
- Hydronephrosis

Management
The patient should be referred to the urology department for pain management, hydration and extracorporeal shock wave lithotripsy (ESWL). If the calculus is causing hydronephrosis and

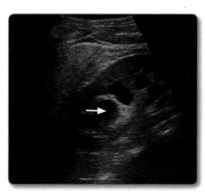

Figure 5.9 Ultrasound of a left kidney demonstrates dilatation of the pelvicaliceal system (arrow) due to obstruction by a ureteric calculus.

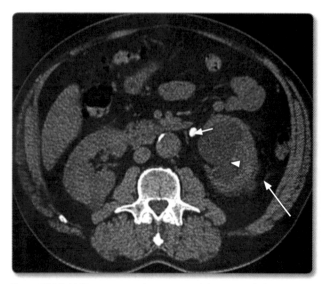

Figure 5.10 Axial CT non-contrast demonstrates a left ureteric calculus (arrow) resulting in hydroneprosis of the left kidney (arrowhead) and surrounding perinephric stranding (long arrow).

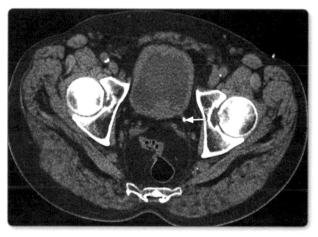

Figure 5.11 Axial CT non-contrast demonstrates a left distal ureteric calculus at the vesico-ureteric junction (arrow).

complicated by infection, the patient may require a percutaneous nephrostomy and opinion on interventional radiology should be sought.

5.5 Testicular torsion

Testicular torsion results from twisting of the spermatic cord, strangulation of blood flow and resulting ischaemia and infarction of the testis. The majority of patients affected are adolescents and young men.

Key facts

- The differential diagnosis for an acute scrotum includes: torsion of the testis or testicular appendix, epididymo-orchitis, testicular hematoma secondary to trauma and an incarcerated scrotal hernia
- Ultrasound can be used to differentiate from other causes of acute scrotum and when the clinical signs are equivocal for torsion

Clinical insight

Testicular torsion salvage rates are nearly 100% in the first 6 hours, 70% between 6 and 12 hours, and 20% between 12 and 24 hours. Therefore, suspected testicular torsion needs emergency surgical exploration, and this should not be delayed for any reason, including imaging. Time is crucial.

Radiographic findings

US The testis may demonstrate normal homogenous echogenicity in the early stages of torsion. However, as there is increased ischaemia of the testis, ultrasound will demonstrate heterogeneous echogenicity. In testicular infarction, hypoechoic areas are demonstrated within the testis.

Colour Doppler This can be used to demonstrate blood flow in the testis and surrounding scrotal structures. However, normal flow may also be seen in testicular torsion and so is not a specific finding. Hence, a normal testicular ultrasound does not exclude a testicular torsion.

Findings of testicular infarction are an enlarged testis with heterogenous echogenicity and areas of hypoechogenicity, absence of blood flow and hydrocoele (**Figure 5.12**).

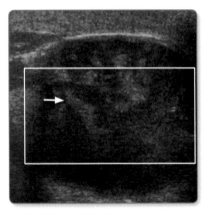

Figure 5.12 Ultrasound of an infarcted testis demonstrates heterogenous echogenicity and testicular enlargement, with no colour flow (arrow) due to a testicular torsion.

Key signs
- Normal ultrasound that does not exclude torsion
- Heterogeneous echogenicity
- Reduction/absence of colour flow

Management
If testicular torsion is suspected, the patient should undergo emergency surgical exploration without any delay.

5.6 Ovarian torsion

Ovarian torsion may be due to partial or complete rotation of the ovary on its vascular pedicle, resulting in ischaemia. Patients commonly present with sharp iliac fossa pain, nausea and vomiting, fever and, on examination, there may be a palpable abdominal mass. Patients will frequently present with non-specific symptoms making the diagnosis difficult, so a high index of suspicion is required.

Key facts
- Ovarian torsion commonly occurs in patients with ovarian cysts or masses
- Adnexal torsion is used to describe twisting of the ovary, fallopian tube or both

Radiographic findings

US Ultrasound is the modality of choice when assessing for ovarian torsion. Direct comparison with the normal side can help. On the affected side the ovary may be enlarged with peripheral follicles. The twisted vascular pedicle may be demonstrated with a 'whirlpool' sign on colour Doppler. Colour Doppler will demonstrate reduced or absent flow within the ovary. However, the presence of colour flow does not allow exclude torsion. There can be free fluid within the pelvis/pouch of Douglas.

Key signs
- Enlarged ovary (**Figure 5.13**)
- Peripheral follicles
- Twisted vascular pedicle with 'whirlpool' sign
- Reduced/absence of colour flow
- Free fluid in pelvis

Management

The patient should be referred to the gynaecological team for emergency laparoscopy/laparotomy. If the ovary is infarcted, then an oophrectomy will be performed.

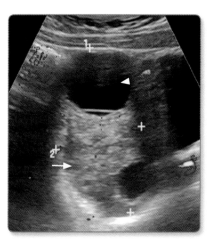

Figure 5.13 Ultrasound of an enlarged ovarian torsion (arrow). The large cystic structure is a twisted fallopian tube (arrowhead). Power Doppler demonstrates no flow within the ovary.

Chest and vascular disease

6.1 Key radiological anatomy

Lungs and pleural cavity

Lungs

The lungs are divided into lobes by fissures (**Figures 6.1–6.5**).
The right lung Ⓐ has three lobes: the upper Ⓑ, middle Ⓒ

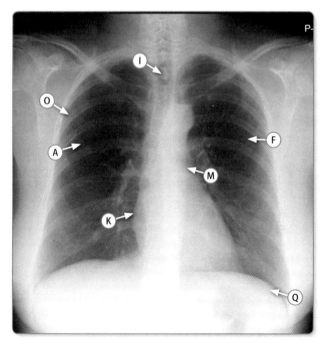

Figure 6.1 Chest radiograph demonstrating the right lung Ⓐ, left lung Ⓕ, trachea Ⓘ, heart Ⓚ, descending aorta Ⓜ, rib Ⓞ and diaphragm Ⓠ.

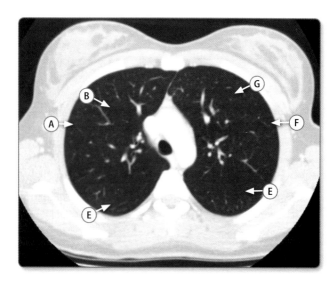

Figure 6.2 Axial CT (lung window) demonstrating right lung Ⓐ, right upper lobe Ⓑ, oblique fissures Ⓔ, left lung Ⓕ and left upper lobe Ⓖ.

and lower Ⓓ lobes, separated by the horizontal and oblique Ⓔ fissures. The left lung Ⓕ has two lobes: the upper Ⓖ and lower Ⓗ, separated by the oblique fissure. Each lobe is further subdivided into bronchopulmonary segments, supplied by a segmental artery, vein and bronchus.

Pleural cavity

The pleura consist of a parietal pleura, lining the mediastinum and thoracic cavity, and the visceral pleura covering the lungs. The pleural cavity is a potential space between the two layers, where fluid, air and pus can accumulate in certain pathologies.

Mediastinum

The mediastinum is the space between the lungs and the pleura. It can be subdivided into the superior, anterior, middle and posterior mediastinum. The mediastinum contains the trachea Ⓘ, oesophagus Ⓙ, thoracic duct, lymph nodes, thymus,

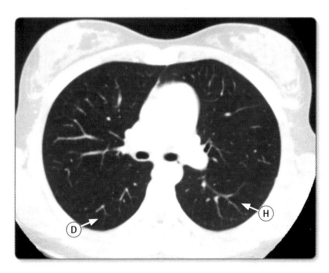

Figure 6.3 Axial CT (lung window) shows the right Ⓓ and left Ⓗ lower lobes of the lung.

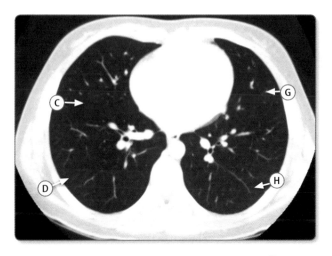

Figure 6.4 Axial CT (lung window) demonstrates right middle lobe Ⓒ, right lower lobe Ⓓ left upper lobe Ⓖ and left lower lobe Ⓗ.

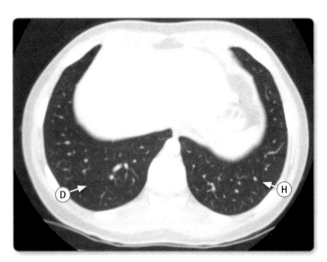

Figure 6.5 Axial CT (lung window) demonstrates the lung bases, right lower lobe Ⓓ and left lower lobe Ⓗ.

heart Ⓚ, great vessels Ⓛ and descending aorta Ⓜ (**Figures 6.1 and 6.6–6.9**).

Thoracic cage

The thoracic cage is formed by 12 thoracic vertebrae Ⓝ, 12 pairs of ribs Ⓞ, the sternum Ⓟ and muscles including the diaphragm Ⓠ (**Figures 6.1** and **6.6–6.9**). The thoracic cage protects as well as aiding inspiration and expiration.

6.2 Thoracic trauma

Thoracic trauma can lead to serious and life-threatening injuries, disrupting ventilation (trauma to the lungs) and perfusion (trauma to the heart and great vessels).

Pneumothorax

Pneumothorax is the accumulation of air in the pleural cavity, which can be spontaneous or the result of blunt or penetrating trauma.

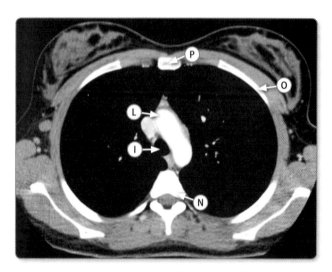

Figure 6.6 Axial CT demonstrates trachea (I), great vessels (L), thoracic vertebra (N), rib (O) and sternum (P).

Key facts

A traumatic pneumothorax commonly occurs due to pulmonary laceration from a sudden rise in intrathoracic pressure, a rib fracture or from penetrating trauma.

A spontaneous pneumothorax results from the rupture of subpleural blebs, commonly seen in smokers.

Radiographic findings

Plain radiograph On an erect chest radiograph, a pneumothorax is demonstrated by visualising the visceral pleura as a sharp line. There is an absence of vascular lung markings beyond this line (**Figure 6.10a**). It is more difficult to visualise a pneumothorax on

Clinical insight

Tension pneumothorax can be fatal as significant mediastinal shift obstructs venous return to the heart. This is a clinical emergency needing prompt decompression. Clinical signs of tension pneumothorax include absent breath sounds and resonance to percussion with tracheal deviation to the contralateral side.

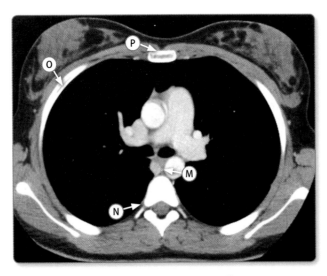

Figure 6.7 Axial CT demonstrates the descending aorta Ⓜ, thoracic vertebra Ⓝ, rib Ⓞ and sternum Ⓟ.

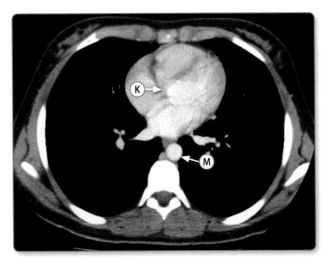

Figure 6.8 Axial CT demonstrates the heart Ⓚ and descending aorta Ⓜ.

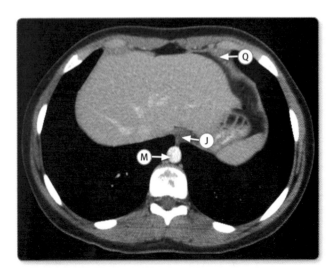

Figure 6.9 Axial CT demonstrates the oesophagus Ⓙ, descending aorta Ⓜ and diaphragm Ⓠ.

a supine chest radiograph as the air collects anterior to the lungs. Subtle signs of pneumothorax on supine radiographs include a sharp well-demarcated mediastinal border or a 'deep sulcus sign'.

Mediastinal shift can be seen on a chest radiograph as the trachea deviates to the contralateral side.

CT Computed tomography (CT) will demonstrate the pneumothorax, as well as other injuries sustained and causative factors (e.g. rib fractures, foreign body).

Key signs
- Sharply demarcated visceral pleura on erect chest radiograph
- Deep sulcus sign on supine chest radiograph
- Mediastinal shift
- Rib fractures

Management
Further management of the patient will depend on the size of the pneumothorax and the patient's symptomatology. If there

is a large pneumothorax then a chest drain should be inserted (**Figure 6.10b**).

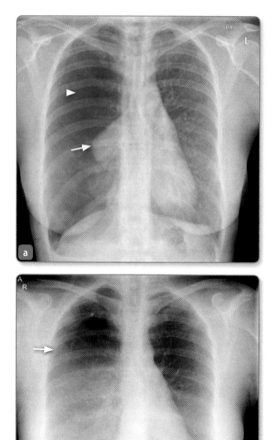

Figure 6.10 (a) Chest X-ray demonstrating a right-sided pneumothorax. The visceral surface of the lung is seen (arrow) with absence of vascular markings (arrowhead). (b) Chest X-ray after insertion of a chest drain (arrow). The lung has started to reinflate.

Haemothorax

Haemothorax is the accumulation of blood in the pleural cavity.

Key facts
- Haemothorax can result from penetrating or blunt trauma, surgery or interventional procedures, such as thoracocentesis
- A small haemothorax occurs due to lung contusions and lacerations, resulting in blood accumulating from low-pressure pulmonary circulation
- A life-threatening, larger haemothorax arises from injury to systemic or large pulmonary vessels. Due to significant haemorrhage, patients will develop hypovolaemic shock and need to be resuscitated

Radiographic findings

Plain radiograph On a posteroanterior (PA) view, the first 300 ml of blood within the pleural space may not be visualised as the blood accumulates in the subpulmonic region. In a massive haemothorax, there is enlargement of the ipsilateral hemithorax, with displacement of the mediastinum to the contralateral side (**Figure 6.11a**). On supine radiograph, the haemothorax will accumulate posteriorly, resulting in a diffuse increase in density on the affected side.

CT CT will demonstrate the haemothorax, as well as possible underlying causes and associated injuries.

Key signs
- 'White out' and meniscus appearance
- Mediastinal shift to the contralateral side
- Diffuse increase in density on supine radiograph
- Injury to great vessels or pulmonary vessels

Management
Patients with a massive haemothorax will need to be transferred to a thoracic surgical unit. A large bore chest drain should be inserted, with caution as there is a risk of exsanguination (**Figure 6.11b**).

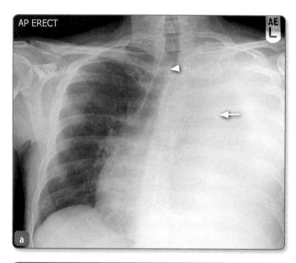

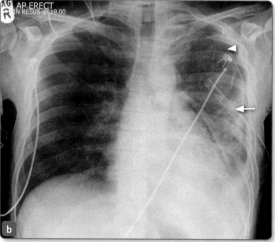

Figure 6.11 (a) Chest X-ray demonstrating a large left haemothorax with complete 'white out' of the lung (arrow) with mediastinal shift to the right (arrowhead). (b) Chest X-ray after insertion of a chest drain (arrow). There is a small left pneumothorax (arrowhead).

Flail chest

Flail chest results from fractures of three or more adjacent ribs in two places, or adjacent sternum, rib or costochondral fractures. The flail segment results in impaired ventilation as it moves paradoxically to the rest of the thoracic cage.

Key facts

- A flail segment may be clinically obvious, as a portion of the chest wall moves paradoxically to the rest of the chest wall
- Severe pulmonary contusions (intra-alveolar and interstitial haemorrhage) and other intrathoracic injuries are seen in patients with flail chest

Radiographic findings

Plain radiograph Plain radiograph will demonstrate multiple rib fractures, pulmonary contusions (**Figure 6.12**) and associated haemothorax and pneumothoraces. There may be extensive subcutaneous emphysema due to the rib fractures and air leak (**Figure 6.13**).

CT CT will confirm a flail segment (with rib fractures at two sites in multiple ribs). CT will also allow assessment of other injuries sustained (**Figure 6.14**).

Key signs

- Multiple rib fractures, in two places
- Pulmonary contusion
- Haemothorax, pneumothorax
- Subcutaneous emphysema

Management

The aim of management is to protect the lung and to provide adequate ventilation. Adequate analgesia is important in patients who have sustained rib fractures, and there may be a role for a local nerve block in patients with a flail chest.

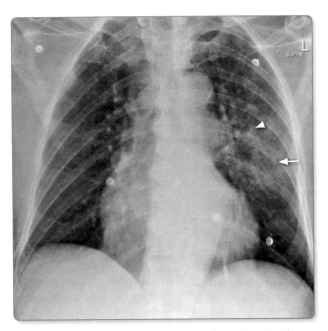

Figure 6.12 Chest X-ray demonstrating left-sided rib fractures (arrow), with underlying pulmonary contusions (arrowhead).

Aortic transection

Aortic injury can be partial or complete. Partial injury results in disruption of the inner layers of the aortic wall. Complete injury results in disruption of all the layers and is usually rapidly fatal.

Key facts

- There is a focal transverse tear of the aorta at the site of relative fixation, i.e. isthmus (ligamentum arteriosum), root and diaphragm
- Approximately 90% of aortic transection occurs at the isthmus (distal to the origin of the left subclavian artery)
- Aortic injury can result in false aneurysm formation, focal dissection, intramural haematoma and massive exsanguinations, and death

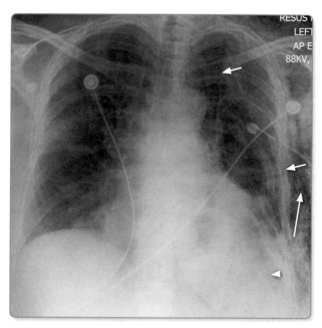

Figure 6.13 Chest X-ray demonstrating multiple left-sided rib fractures with breaks in two parts of the rib (arrows), with a small haemothorax (arrowhead) and subcutaneous emphysema (long arrow).

Radiographic findings

Plain radiograph Plain radiograph will demonstrate a widened mediastinum. The contours of the aortic arch can be blurred with filling of the aortopulmonary window. There can also be a left apical cap due to extra pleural haematoma. Massive haemothorax, pulmonary contusions, pneumothorax and rib injuries may also be demonstrated.

CT CT is the modality to assess the extent of injuries. Aortic injury will be demonstrated as an irregular contour of the descending aorta, focal dissection and intramural haematoma.

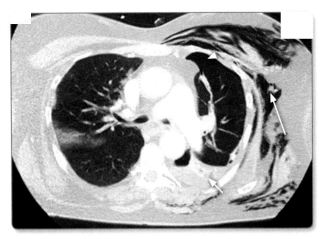

Figure 6.14 Axial CT (lung window) demonstrating a small haemothorax (arrow), with a small pneumothorax (arrowhead) and subcutaneous emphysema (long arrow).

Key signs
- Widened mediastinum
- Apical cap
- Aortic transection, dissection, aneurysm (**Figure 6.15**)
- Haemothorax/pulmonary contusions

Management
Aortic transection can be managed by endovascular stenting. However, mortality remains high even after repair due to associated synchronous injuries that are also often life-threatening.

6.3 Acute aortic syndrome

Acute aortic syndrome describes thoracic aortic disease encompassing three pathologies: dissection, penetrating ulcer and intramural haematoma.

Key facts
- Penetrating ulcers are usually atherosclerotic in origin. The ulcer penetrates the thrombus and intima into the media.

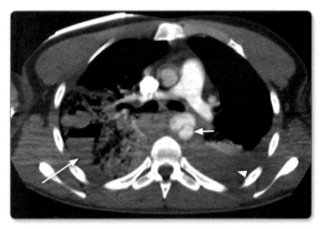

Figure 6.15 Axial CT demonstrating traumatic aortic injury (arrow), with a left pleural effusion (arrowhead) and lung contusions (long arrow).

This can progress to intramural haematoma, dissection, false aneurysm and aortic rupture

- Intramural haematoma occurs due to haemorrhage of the vaso vasorum, with blood extending into the media and tracking along the aorta. This can then develop into a true dissection

- Aortic dissection is longitudinal separation of the aortic intima and adventitia. This has been classified into Stanford A (involves the aortic root and arch) and Stanford B (involves the descending aorta only)

> **Clinical insight**
>
> Patients will present with symptoms (i.e. sudden-onset chest, back or abdominal pain) that can mimic other common conditions. Therefore, a high index of suspicion is required for aortic dissection.

Radiographic findings

Plain radiograph Plain radiograph can be normal. The mediastinum can be widened with associated left pleural effusion. Aortic wall calcification may be displaced inwards from the outer contour, secondary to the dissection.

CT Pre and post contrast CT is the imaging modality of choice to assess aortic dissection. Pre contrast scans will demonstrate intramural haematoma as circumferential high attenuation of the ascending aorta. Post contrast, the true lumen can be differentiated from the false lumen (within the media) (**Figures 6.16–6.18**). The true lumen is invariably the smaller lumen and is confluent with non-involved aortic lumen. This can help to identify potential end-organ complications and aid intervention.

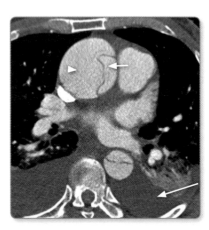

Figure 6.16 Axial CT demonstrating aortic dissection with a true lumen (arrow), larger false lumen (arrowhead) and pleural effusions (long arrow).

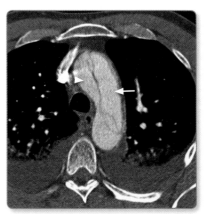

Figure 6.17 Axial CT demonstrating aortic dissection with a true lumen (arrow) and larger false lumen (arrowhead).

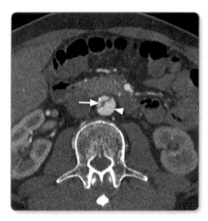

Figure 6.18 Axial CT demonstrating aortic dissection extending into the abdominal aorta, with a true lumen (arrow) and larger false lumen (arrowhead).

Key signs
- Normal chest radiograph
- Widened mediastinum
- Intramural haematoma (**Figure 6.19**)
- Dissection flap
- True and false lumen

Management
Management can be conservative or surgical and will depend on patient factors and the extent of the dissection.

6.4 Abdominal aortic aneurysm

Abdominal aortic aneurysm rupture should be excluded in patients with acute abdominal pain, especially when they present with flank or back pain. Causes of abdominal aortic aneurysm include atherosclerosis, trauma, congenital, infection and inflammation.

Key facts
- The abdominal aorta is generally referred to as aneurysmal when the diameter exceeds 30 mm. A true aneurysm involves all layers of the aortic wall

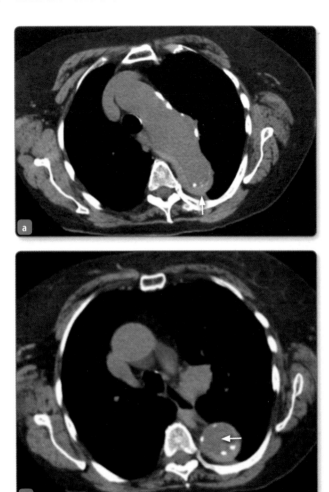

Figure 6.19 (a) Axial CT demonstrating a crescentic high attenuation, in keeping with intramural haematoma (arrow). (b) Axial CT demonstrating intramural haematoma displacing the aortic calcification medially (arrow).

- Risk factors include age more than 75 years, male sex, known ischaemic heart disease, hypertension, smoking and hyper-cholesterolaemia

Radiographic findings

Plain radiograph An incidental finding on plain abdominal radiograph is a calcified abdominal aortic aneurysm (**Figure 6.20**). This should be investigated further with ultrasound (US) or CT.

Clinical insight

One of the most important features of impending or contained rupture in the emergency setting is the presence of a painful aneurysm.

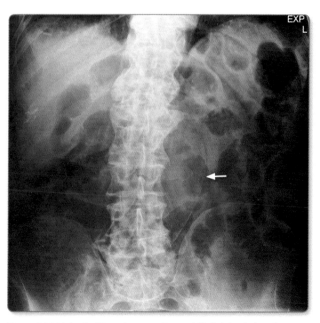

Figure 6.20 Abdominal X-ray demonstrating a calcified abdominal aortic aneurysm (arrow).

CT Features of impending or contained aneurysm rupture include a high attenuation crescent, draping over the spine and focal discontinuity in intimal calcification. A ruptured aneurysm will be demonstrated on both pre and post contrast scans. A large retroperitoneal haematoma will be demonstrated with active extravasation of contrast.

Key signs
- Dilated abdominal aorta >3 mm (**Figure 6.21**)
- Break in aortic calcification and high attenuation crescent
- Large retroperitoneal haematoma (**Figure 6.22**)
- Free intraperitoneal fluid

Management
A patient presenting with a painful abdominal aortic aneurysm requires the consideration of urgent repair. This may be an endovascular repair, if suitable, or conventional surgical repair. In the case of abdominal aortic aneurysm rupture, emergency surgical repair is undertaken.

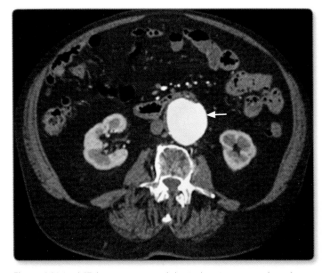

Figure 6.21 Axial CT demonstrating an abdominal aortic aneurysm (arrow).

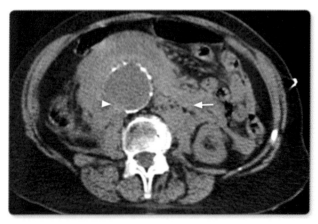

Figure 6.22 Axial CT demonstrating abdominal aortic aneurysm rupture. There is a large retroperitoneal haematoma (arrow) and break in the aortic calcification at the site of rupture (arrowhead).

6.5 Deep vein thrombosis

Deep vein thrombosis (DVT) forms from blood constituents in flowing blood. Patients will present with unilateral leg swelling, tenderness, pain and increased temperature.

Key facts

- Hypercoagulability, venous stasis and vessel injury all predispose to developing a DVT
- Risk factors include recent surgery, trauma, prolonged immobilisation, obesity and malignancy

Radiographic findings

US Ultrasound is the modality of choice to assess for DVT. Ultrasound will demonstrate lack of luminal collapse on compression, due to the presence of thrombus. There may be echogenic thrombus seen within a distended vein. The common femoral vein will not increase in diameter during the Valsava manoeuvre. There will be no flow seen in the obstructed vessel on colour Doppler examination.

Key signs

- Distended vein
- Lack of collapse on compression
- Echogenic luminal thrombus (**Figure 6.23**)

Management

Once a DVT has been confirmed, the patient will require anti-coagulation to prevent pulmonary embolism.

6.6 Pulmonary embolism

Pulmonary embolism (PE) can be fatal if the diagnosis is delayed or missed. Patients typically presents with pleuritic chest pain, acute shortness of breath and haemoptysis.

Key facts

- Embolism commonly results from leg DVT, which travels to the right side of the heart and into the pulmonary arteries

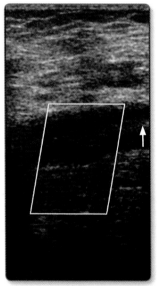

Figure 6.23 Ultrasound of deep vein demonstrating an echogenic thrombus within a distended vein (arrow). No colour flow is demonstrated.

- Pulmonary embolism can result in right heart strain, dysfunction and failure, leading to circulatory collapse and death

Radiographic findings

Nuclear medicine Ventilation/perfusion scans can be used to determine the probability of PE in patients who have a normal chest radiograph with no known underlying cardiac or respiratory disease. A PE will be demonstrated as a hypoperfused segment of lung which has normal ventilation. Findings of the ventilation and perfusion scan need correlation with the clinical probability of PE.

CT A CT pulmonary angiogram will demonstrate filling defects within the pulmonary arteries. The main, lobar, segmental as well as subsegmental pulmonary arteries need to be evaluated. CT will also demonstrate peripheral wedge lung infarcts and oedema. There can be signs of right heart strain, including increased main pulmonary artery diameter and straightening of the intraventicular septum.

Key signs
- Perfusion defect in a normally ventilated lung segment
- Luminal filling defects on CT (**Figure 6.24**)
- Evidence of right heart strain

Management
Management will depend on the severity of PE and associated complications. There may be a role for thrombolysis in severe life-threatening cases. The majority of patients will be started on anticoagulants.

6.7 Foreign bodies

Foreign bodies can be inhaled or ingested. Depending on the level of obstruction, an inhaled foreign body is a medical emergency, needing rapid assessment and treatment. Commonly, children will present with an episode of coughing, wheezing or choking, while eating or playing.

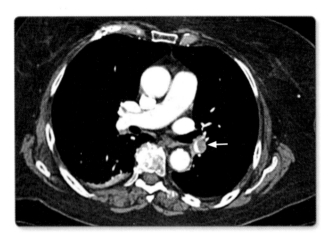

Figure 6.24 Axial CT demonstrating pulmonary emboli as filling defects in the left pulmonary arteries (arrow).

Key facts

- If the obstruction is lower than the main bronchus, patients will present with persistent wheeze, cough and dyspnoea. There may be persistent or recurrent pneumonia, or the child may be asymptomatic
- Blunt ingested foreign bodies (i.e. coins) can lodge in the oesophagus, leading to mucosal erosion. In such cases, a single chest radiograph is indicated to confirm the position of the foreign body
- The location of sharp and poisonous (e.g. batteries) foreign bodies always needs to be confirmed because of the risk of perforation due to mucosal damage. This requires both chest and abdominal radiographs
- Batteries can result in the leak of caustic substances leading to mucosal erosion and perforation and will need emergency removal via endoscopy if lodged in the oesophagus

Radiographic findings

Plain radiograph Plain radiograph will demonstrate radio-opaque foreign bodies and the level of obstruction (**Figures 6.25**

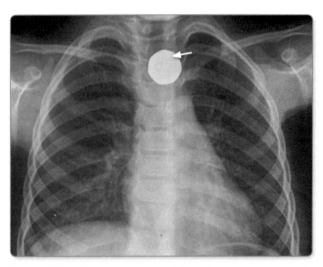

Figure 6.25 Chest X-ray demonstrating a coin lodged in the oesophagus (arrow).

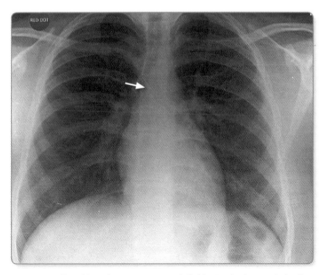

Figure 6.26 Chest X-ray demonstrating an inhaled foreign body: a pin lodged in the carina, extending into the left main bronchus (arrow).

and **6.26**). If the foreign body has been inhaled, there may be air trapping on the affected side on expiration.

Management

The majority of ingested foreign bodies will pass and be excreted without the need for intervention. Ingested batteries need urgent removal to prevent oesophageal injury from caustic leak. Depending on the level of obstruction for inhaled foreign bodies, emergency treatment in the form of paediatric life support resuscitation for an upper airway obstruction should be carried out. Lower airway obstruction will require surgery for removal.

chapter 7

Head and neck

7.1 Key radiological anatomy

Facial bones

Patients with facial trauma will be initially assessed and, if necessary, plain radiographs will be requested. Two views are usually obtained as part of a trauma series: occipitomental (OM) 15 and OM 30 views. On an OM 15 view (**Figure 7.1**) structures to review are the frontal bone Ⓐ, frontal sinuses Ⓑ, zygomatic bone Ⓒ, maxilla Ⓓ, maxillary sinuses Ⓔ and mandible Ⓕ. Indirect signs of injury include overlying soft tissue swelling and fluid levels within the sinuses.

Common facial fractures disrupt the three 'Lines of Dolan' (**Figure 7.2**), which when drawn can look like elephant trunks:

1. The **orbital line** ⓄⓁ is drawn through the zygomaticofrontal suture, along the superior orbital rim and through the frontal sinuses
2. The **zygomatic line** ⓏⓁ is drawn along the superior border of the zygomatic arch, the inferior orbital rim and over the nasal bridge
3. The **maxillary line** ⓂⓁ is along the inferior border of the zygomatic arch, inferior margins of maxillary antra and across the maxilla

Mandible

Mandibular injuries can be assessed on an orthopantomogram (OPT). The mandible consists of a body Ⓖ, angle Ⓗ, ramus Ⓘ, condyle Ⓙ and coronoid process Ⓚ (**Figure 7.3**). The temporomandibular (TM) joint Ⓛ comprises the mandibular condyle and the articular tubercle of the temporal bone.

Orbits

Computed tomography (CT) is the modality of choice to assess bony injury to the orbit (**Figure 7.4**). Bony structures to

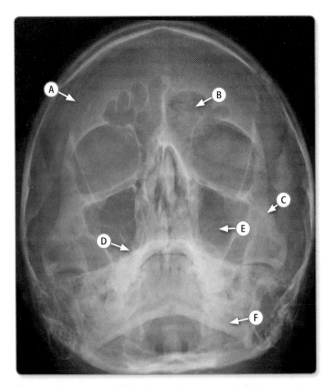

Figure 7.1 Occipito-mental (OM) 15 view demonstrating the facial bones and sinuses. Frontal bone (A), frontal sinuses (B), zygomatic bone (C), maxilla (D), maxillary sinuses (E) and mandible (F).

assess include the orbital roof (M), medial orbital wall (N) lateral orbital wall (O) and the orbital floor (P). Important soft tissue structures that are assessed better by magnetic resonance imaging (MRI) include the optic nerve (Q), inferior rectus muscle (R), lateral rectus muscle (S), medial rectus muscle (T) and superior rectus muscle (U) (**Figures 7.4** to **7.6**).

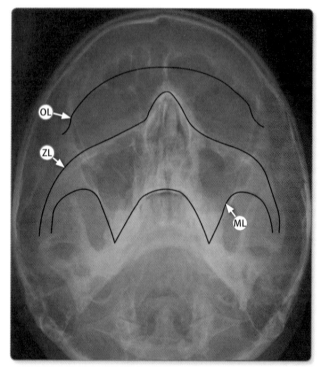

Figure 7.2 Occipitomental (OM) 30 view demonstrating the lines of Dolan. Orbital line (OL), zygomatic line (ZL) and maxillary line (ML).

Soft tissues of the neck

The deep spaces of the suprahyoid head and neck contain fascial-bound compartments within which infection can track and spread beyond (**Figure 7.7**).

These spaces include the:

- **Masticator space** (v): this is lateral to the parapharyngeal space and contains the muscles of mastication, ramus and body of mandible, and the mandibular division of the trigeminal nerve

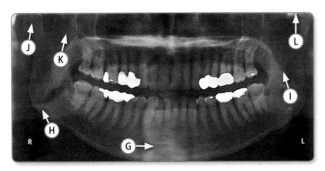

Figure 7.3 Orthopanto-mogram demonstrating the mandible anatomy: Body Ⓖ, angle Ⓗ, ramus Ⓘ, condyle Ⓙ, coronoid process Ⓚ and the temporo mandibular joint Ⓛ.

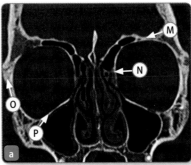

Figure 7.4 (a) Coronal CT scan showing the bony structure of the orbits. Orbital roof Ⓜ, medial orbital wall Ⓝ, lateral orbital wall Ⓞ and the orbital floor Ⓟ. (b) Coronal CT scan showing the soft tissue structures of the orbits. Optic nerve Ⓠ, inferior rectus muscle Ⓡ, lateral rectus muscle Ⓢ, medial rectus muscle Ⓣ and superior rectus muscle Ⓤ.

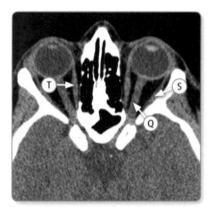

Figure 7.5 Axial CT scan showing the optic nerve Ⓠ, lateral rectus Ⓢ and medial rectus Ⓣ.

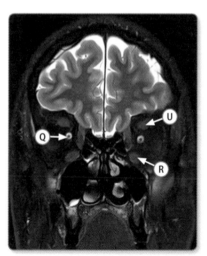

Figure 7.6 Coronal MR T2-weighted scan demonstrating the optic nerve Ⓠ, superior rectus Ⓤ and inferior rectus Ⓡ.

- **Parapharyngeal space** Ⓦ: this is a centrally located space extending from the skull base to the hyoid. This space is effaced when there are lesions within the other spaces (**Table 7.1** and **Figure 7.8**)

- **Retropharyngeal space** ⓧ: this is a potential space anterior to the prevertebral space, extending from the skull base to the third thoracic vertebra

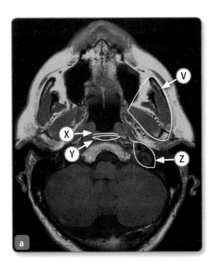

Figure 7.7 (a) Axial MR at the level of the nasopharynx demonstrating the masticator space ⓥ, retropharyngeal space ⓧ, prevertebral space ⓨ and carotid space ⓩ. (b) Axial MR at the level of the oropharynx demonstrating the masticator space ⓥ, parapharyngeal space ⓦ, retropharyngeal space ⓧ, prevertebral space ⓨ and parotid space ⒶⒶ.

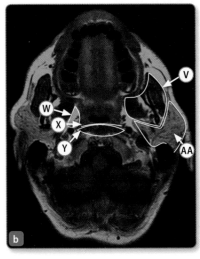

Compartment in which pathology present	Direction in which parapharyngeal space is effaced
Masticator space	Posteromedial
Retropharyngeal space	Anterolateral
Carotid space	Anterior
Parotid space	Anteromedial

Table 7.1 Effacement of the parapharyngeal space by pathologies in related deep spaces of the suprahyoid head and neck.

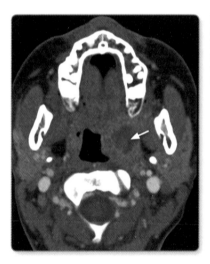

Figure 7.8 Axial CT post contrast demonstrating a large left parapharyngeal abscess (arrow) with displacement of the oropharynx.

- **Prevertebral space** Ⓨ: this is a space posterior to the retropharyngeal space extending from the skull base to the fourth thoracic vertebra
- **Carotid space** Ⓩ: This composes the carotid fascia which extends from the skull base to the aortic arch
- **Parotid space** ⒶⒶ: This space contains the parotid gland, facial nerve and the retromandibular vein

7.2 Facial trauma

Facial injury and fractures are common presentations in the emergency department as a result of road traffic collisions, assault, falls and other trauma. The type of injury sustained depends upon the part of the face injured and the force applied.

Localised injuries (**Figures 7.9-7.11**) include nasoethmoid fractures, zygomatic complex fractures, mid facial fractures and mandibular fractures.

Key facts

- A naso-orbito-ethmoid (NOE) complex fracture results from trauma to the nasal bridge. The fracture extends into the nose through the ethmoids and is more serious than isolated nasal bone fracture
- Zygomatico complex fracture (tripod): this includes fractures through the zygomaticofrontal, zygomaticotemporal and zygomaticomaxillary sutures. It is essential to assess involvement of the orbital floor as this affects management of the patient
- Mid-facial fractures include LeFort I, II and III fractures – these result in separation of part or all of a portion of the maxilla from the skull base. In order to be classed as a Le

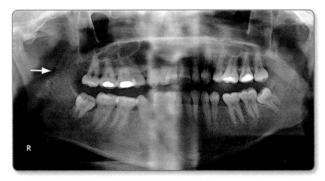

Figure 7.9 Orthopantomogram demonstrating a right-sided mandibular fracture (arrow).

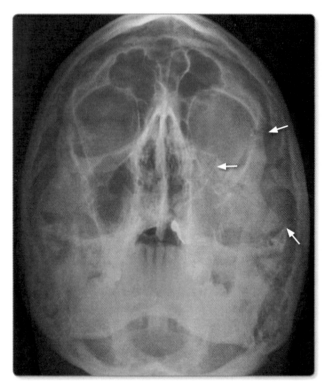

Figure 7.10 Facial radiograph demonstrating a left zygomatic complex fracture and disruption in the Lines of Dolan (arrows).

Fort fracture, the junction of the posterior maxillary sinus with the pterygoid plates of the sphenoid must be disrupted
- The mandible is considered an incomplete ring and hence fractures usually involve both sides of the mandible. Therefore, if one fracture is observed another should be sought. Mandibular fractures can be associated with TM joint dislocation
- Complex mid facial and mandibular fractures can compromise the airway and hence it should be secured before imaging

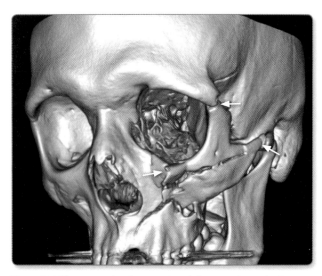

Figure 7.11 CT reconstruction demonstrating a left zygomatic complex fracture.

Radiographic findings

Plain radiograph Direct signs of facial fracture include disruptions of the Dolan lines. These may be seen as linear lucencies, cortical defects, bone fragments overlying each other and facial asymmetry. Indirect signs include soft tissue swelling and fluid levels in the paranasal sinuses.

CT CT is the modality of choice and the signs seen on plain radiographs are better appreciated. Another subtle sign that a fracture is present includes intracranial or intraorbital air.

Key signs
- Disruption of lines of Dolan
- Intraorbital air
- Mandibular instability

Management
Further management of the patient will depend on the severity of the injury sustained and its location. Referral to

ear, nose and throat (ENT) or maxillofacial surgeons should be made.

7.3 Orbital trauma

Orbital fractures are usually the result of direct trauma to the orbit.

Key facts

- 'Blowout' fractures of the orbital wall are the result of blunt trauma. The term 'blowout' is used when there is a fracture of the inferior (floor) and/or medial wall of the orbit and the orbital rim is intact

> **Clinical insight**
>
> Make sure to examine eye movements in a patient who has sustained a blow to the orbit. Restriction of upward gaze indicates an associated injury to the inferior rectus muscle. Loss of vision or decreasing visual acuity warrants urgent ophthalmology referral.

- Inferior wall or floor fracture may occur in combination with other facial fractures. This includes posterior extension of the zygomatico complex fracture into the zygomatico sphenoid suture (quadripod). Le Fort II fractures also involve the orbital floor. NOE complex fractures can involve the medial wall
- High impact fractures of the brain and cervical spine can involve the superior orbital rim, part of the frontal bone. Involvement of the posterior wall of the frontal sinus can result in cerebrospinal fluid (CSF) rhinorrhoea and possibly meningitis

Radiographic findings

Plain radiograph An orbital floor fracture may be very subtle on plain radiograph and may be interpreted as normal. However, there are indirect signs of orbital floor fracture (**Figure 7.12**), which include fluid level in the maxillary sinus and overlying soft tissue swelling. There may be additional soft tissue seen under the orbital floor 'teardrop sign'. This indicates herniation of intraorbital fat and the inferior rectus muscle through the orbital floor fracture.

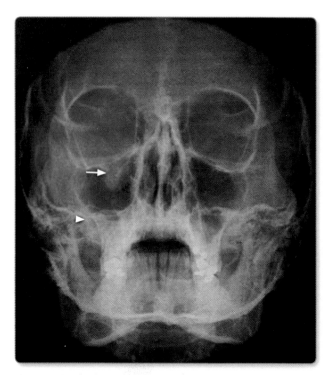

Figure 7.12 Facial radio-graph demonstrating a right orbital floor fracture and teardrop sign (arrow) with fluid level in the maxillary sinus (arrowhead).

CT This will demonstrate the extent of injury and related complications including retrobulbar haematoma, optic nerve injury and injury to the muscles.

Key signs
- Disruption of orbital walls, floor, roof (**Figures 7.13a** and **b**)
- Opacification of maxillary sinuses
- Herniation and thickening of recti muscles/orbital fat (**Figure 7.13c**)

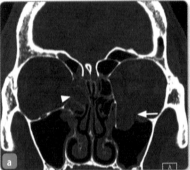

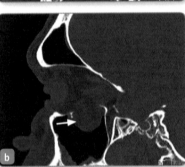

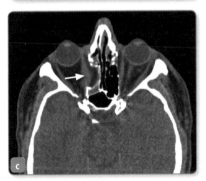

Figure 7.13 (a) Coronal CT demonstrating a left orbital floor fracture and herniation of the inferior rectus and orbital fat into the maxillary sinus (arrow). There is a right medial orbital wall fracture (arrowhead). (b) Sagittal CT demonstrating a left orbital floor fracture and herniation of the inferior rectus and orbital fat into the maxillary sinus (arrow). (c) Axial CT demonstrating a right medial orbital wall fracture and herniation and thickening of the medial rectus (arrow).

Management

- Urgent surgery is indicated if a fracture fragment is imping-ing on the optic nerve/canal or if a retrobulbar haemorrhage is present
- Management of orbital wall fracture is based on clinical and radiological evaluation and will guide whether, when or how to repair the fracture

7.4 Orbital infection

Orbital infection commonly results from bacterial infection extending from the paranasal sinuses. Acute infection of the orbit may be confined to the tissues anterior to the orbital septum or extend into the post septal compartment including the extra- and intraconal space. This can lead to subperiosteal or orbital abscess formation and cavernous sinus thrombosis.

Key facts

- Orbital infection is described in relation to the orbital septum as either pre septal (periorbital) or post septal (orbital)
- Distinguishing between the two is clinically very important as post septal infections can result in significant complica-tions, including meningitis and cavernous sinus throm-bosis, that require aggressive treatment

Clinical insight

A patient presenting with preseptal infection will have an oedematous and red eyelid. The eye itself will not be involved. In comparison, a patient presenting with post septal infection will have eyelid signs as well as proptosis, chemosis and diplopia from opthalmoplegia. Late findings include decreased visual acuity.

Radiographic findings

CT Pre and post contrast CT is the modality of choice for assessing orbital infections and their complications. This will demonstrate thickening and oedema of the orbital soft tissues. Post contrast there will be an enhancing collection with a low attenuation rim (**Figure 7.14a**). A subperiosteal abscess will result in lateral displace-ment of the rectus muscle and orbital fat (**Figure 7.14b**).

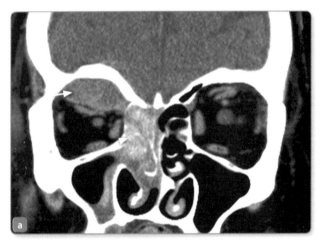

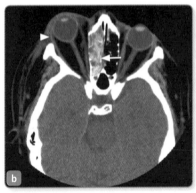

Figure 7.14 (a) Coronal CT demonstrating a collection (arrow) with adjacent ethmoid sinus disease (arrowhead). (b) Axial CT demonstrating an enhancing infection within the right ethmoid air cells (arrow). There is associated proptosis of the right orbit (arrowhead).

Key signs
- Enhancing pre septal/post septal collection
- Subperiosteal abscess
- Intracranial extension
- Cavernous sinus thrombosis
- Paranasal sinus disease

Management

Any patient presenting with orbital infection needs accurate clinical assessment, urgent ophthalmology review and appropriate imaging.

7.5 Retropharyngeal abscess

Retropharyngeal abscess occurs in children as a result of upper respiratory tract infections, tonsillar infection, suppuration of an infected lymph node, perforating injuries of the pharynx or oesophagus, and rarely from cervical discitis. Clinical presentation includes dysphagia, fever and neck stiffness. Narrowing of the pharyngeal lumen can result in stridor.

Key facts

- The retropharyngeal space is posterior to the pharyngeal mucosal space and anterior to the prevertebral space. It extends inferiorly up to the T3 level. Hence, the chest should be included in the imaging protocol
- There will be thickening of the retropharyngeal space, with anterolateral effacement of the parapharyngeal space
- There will be widening of the prevertebral soft tissue shadow on a lateral cervical spine radiograph, confirmed on CT. Normal measurements of prevertebral soft tissue on lateral radiographs of the neck are less than 6 mm at C2 level (any age), less than 14 mm (children) and less than 22 mm at C6 level

Radiographic findings

CT

- Thickening of the retropharyngeal space with fluid collection and frank abscess formation
- This can be associated with pockets of air – either within the abscess or adjacent to it

Key signs

- Widening of the prevertebral soft tissue shadow on a lateral neck radiograph (**Figure 7.15**)

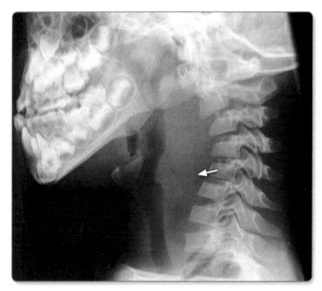

Figure 7.15 Lateral soft tissue neck X-ray demonstrating widening of prevertebral soft tissues (arrow).

- Fluid and/or air in the retropharyngeal compartment on CT
- Extension of the infection into the superior mediastinum

Management
- Immediate airway management and intravenous (IV) antibiotics
- Surgical drainage if the abscess is large and complex

7.6 Foreign bodies

There will be a history of swallowing a foreign body and subsequent dysphagia or odynophagia.

Key facts
- Foreign bodies can be radiolucent (food, plastic, wood) or radio-opaque (coins, pins, needles)

- Bones tend to lodge in the cervical oesophagus at C6 level
- Look for indirect signs of radiolucent foreign body including widening of the prevertebral soft tissue shadow and air

Radiographic findings

Plain radiograph

- Bone ingestion – linear or slightly curved density, particularly at C6 level (**Figure 7.16**)
- Coins and pins – metal density
- Widening of the prevertebral soft tissue shadow

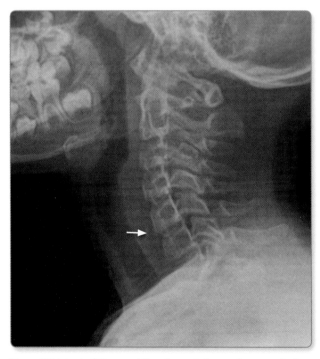

Figure 7.16 Lateral soft tissue neck X-ray demonstrating a radio-opaque foreign body at C5 level in keeping with a fish bone (arrow).

Management
- Most foreign bodies pass down and are excreted
- Impacted bones can be removed by endoscopy
- Button batteries need urgent removal to prevent oesophageal injury from caustic leak

Neurological imaging

8.1 Key radiological anatomy

Skull base and soft tissues

Computed tomography (CT) is the modality of choice when reviewing bone (**Figure 8.1**). Start from the skull base and look for signs of fracture. Indirect signs include soft tissue swelling overlying bone, pneumocephalus and air fluid levels in the sphenoid sinus Ⓐ and mastoid air cells Ⓑ. The sphenoid sinuses and mastoid air cells are normally pneumatised and hence air-filled. A fluid level in either of these structures is suspicious of a skull base fracture. Remember that sinus disease can also present with air fluid level.

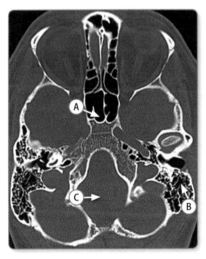

Figure 8.1 Axial CT of skull base in bone window demonstrating the sphenoid sinus Ⓐ, mastoid air cells Ⓑ and foramen magnum Ⓒ.

Posterior cranial fossa

The posterior cranial fossa (**Figures 8.2** and **8.3**) contains the cerebellum Ⓔ, pons Ⓕ and medulla oblongata. The medulla is continuous with the spinal cord Ⓓ and exits through the foramen magnum Ⓒ. Raised intracranial pressure can lead to cerebellar tonsillar herniation through this foramen (coning).

The basilar artery is seen anterior to the pons Ⓖ. Thrombosis and aneurysm are common pathologies associated with the basilar artery.

The cerebral hemispheres

The cerebral hemispheres and basal ganglia structures occupy the supratentorial cranial cavity (**Figures 8.4–8.6**). Each cerebral hemisphere is divided into four lobes: frontal Ⓗ, temporal Ⓘ, parietal Ⓙ and occipital Ⓚ.

Ventricles and basal cisterns

Cerebrospinal fluid (CSF) fills the ventricles, basal cisterns and subarachnoid space of the brain and spinal cord. The ventricles consist of two lateral ventricles Ⓛ (**Figure 8.5**): the midline third Ⓜ, which is connected to the fourth Ⓝ ventricle by the

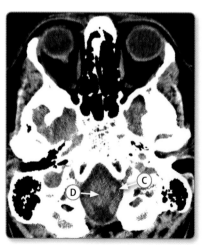

Figure 8.2 Axial CT of skull base in soft tissue window demonstrating the foramen magnum Ⓒ and medulla/spinal cord junction Ⓓ.

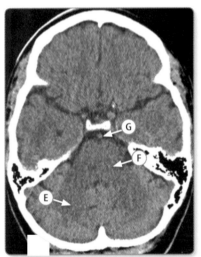

Figure 8.3 Axial CT demonstrating the posterior fossa, containing the cerebellum (E), pons (F) and basilar artery (G).

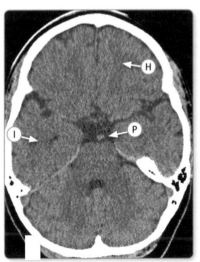

Figure 8.4 Axial CT demonstrating the frontal lobes (H), temporal lobes (I) and suprasellar cistern (P).

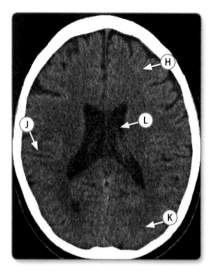

Figure 8.5 Axial CT at the level of lateral ventricles Ⓛ. The frontal Ⓗ parietal Ⓙ and occipital lobes Ⓚ are seen.

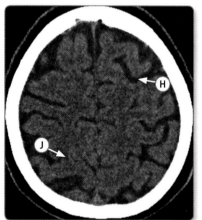

Figure 8.6 Axial CT demonstrating the frontal Ⓗ and parietal lobes. Ⓙ.

cerebral aqueduct Ⓞ (**Figure 8.7**). Basal cisterns are areas at the base of the brain containing CSF Ⓟ (**Figure 8.4**). They are formed by the separation of the arachnoid and pia mater. Raised

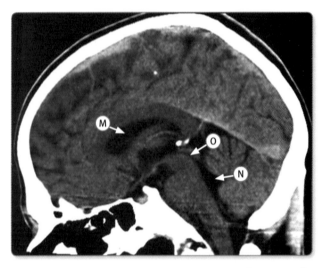

Figure 8.7 Sagittal CT in the midline, demonstrating the third (M) and fourth (N) ventricles and cerebral aqueduct (O).

intracranial pressure and mass effect can lead to compression of the ventricles and effacement of basal cisterns, resulting in obstructive hydrocephalus.

Circle of Willis

The blood supply to the brain (**Figure 8.8**) is derived from the internal carotid (Q) and vertebral arteries (R). The circle of Willis is an anastomosis of the two internal carotid and two vertebral arteries via the basilar artery (R). The anterior cerebral arteries (ACA) supply the superior and medial parts of the brain, including the frontal poles (S). The middle cerebral arteries (MCA) supply the lateral parts of the brain, including the temporal poles (T). The posterior cerebral arteries (PCA) supply the inferior surface of the brain, including the occipital poles (U). Branches from the basilar artery, as well as the terminal portion of the vertebral arteries, supply the posterior fossa structures.

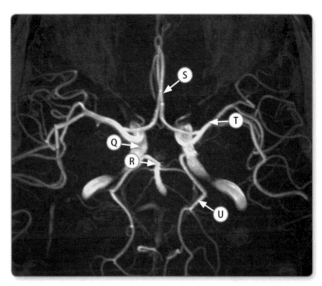

Figure 8.8 A time-of-flight MR angiography image demonstrating the circle of Willis. Internal carotid artery (Q), basilar artery (R), anterior cerebral artery (S), middle cerebral artery (T), posterior cerebral artery (U).

Dural venous sinuses

The dural venous sinuses along with the cortical veins allow venous drainage of the brain (V) (**Figure 8.9**). Major dural sinuses, including the superior, inferior, straight, transverse and sigmoid sinus, drain into the internal jugular veins. The confluence of sinuses (W) is where the superior sagittal sinus, straight sinus and transverse sinus meet.

8.2 Head injury

Head injury accounts for a significant number of attendances at emergency departments worldwide.

Key facts

The type of head injury sustained will depend on the age of the patient and the mechanism of trauma. Common intracranial injuries include:

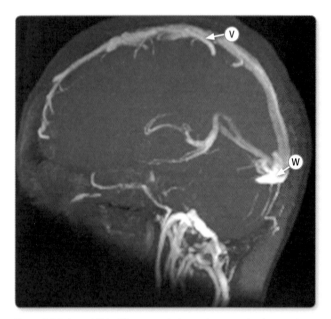

Figure 8.9 A time-of-flight MR venography image demonstrating the superior sagittal sinus (V) and the confluence of sinuses (W).

- Extradural haemorrhage (EDH)
- Subdural haemorrhage (SDH)
- Subarachnoid haemorrhage (SAH)
- Contusions are small focal haemorrhages. These are commonly seen in the inferior, anterior and lateral aspects of the frontal and temporal lobes as the brain moves against the skull base, causing injury.
- Diffuse axonal injury. This results when there is acceleration–deceleration injury to the brain. The gray and white matters are of different densities and will move at different speeds, sliding over one another. As a result, axons that traverse the junction between white and gray matter are stretched.

A patient with a Glasgow Coma Scale (GCS) score of less than 8 will not be able to maintain their airway, and airway adjuncts should be considered (i.e. nasopharyngeal, oropharyngeal airways or intubation). Appropriately trained staff should be available to assess and secure the airway. A patient with significant head injury should be treated with caution as there may be cervical spine injury as well. The neck should be secured before transferring the patient for imaging.

Unenhanced CT head is the first-line investigation to detect haemorrhage, skull fractures and associated complications. The CT scan can appear normal in patients with diffuse axonal injury.

Clinical insight

- When eliciting clinical history, remember the risk factors for sustaining a significant injury, including age of patient, mechanism of injury, vomiting, amnesia, post traumatic seizures and coagulopathy (e.g. is the patient on warfarin?)
- Carry out a full neurological examination and look for signs of skull fracture
- If the history and clinical examination findings meet local guidelines, a CT of the head should be requested urgently

Radiographic findings

CT Acute haemorrhage will present as an area of high attenuation. Large haemorrhaging will cause a mass effect, compressing brain parenchyma, ventricles and basal cisterns, leading to herniation of the brain (**Figure 8.10**). Haemorrhage can also extend into the ventricles, leading to hydrocephalus.

Skull fracture can present with pneumocephalus (intracranial air) (**Figure 8.11**).

Management

Management of the patient will depend on the patient's condition and the nature of the head injury sustained. The care of all patients with abnormal imaging should be discussed with the neurosurgical team.

8.3 Extradural haemorrhage

EDH is typically seen in a young patient with a clear history of head injury. It is usually associated with an underlying skull fracture resulting in arterial bleeding. Accumulation of blood causes mass effect, raised intracranial pressure and decreased GCS. EDH needs urgent neurosurgical input.

Key facts

- Unenhanced CT is the first-line imaging investigation

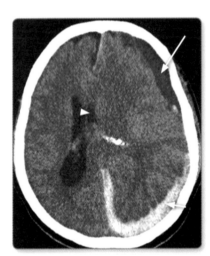

Figure 8.10 CT scan showing acute left subdural haemorrhage (arrow). There is an associated midline shift due to mass effect (arrowhead). There is also a chronic left frontal subdural haemorrhage (long arrow).

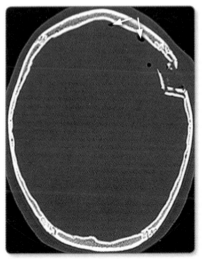

Figure 8.11 CT scan showing pneumocranium (arrows) in the left frontal lobe, due to skull fracture.

Radiographic findings

CT An area of high attenuation on an unenhanced CT scan represents acute haemorrhage. Always look for underlying skull fracture.

It is important to determine the extent of mass effect caused by the haemorrhage.

Key signs
- High attenuation representing acute haemorrhage
- Well-demarcated haemorrhage
- Extra axial and biconvex (**Figure 8.12a**)
- Underlying skull fracture (**Figure 8.12b**)

Management
Urgent neurosurgical referral should be made, irrespective of the size of haemorrhage.

8.4 Subdural haemorrhage

SDH can present acutely in a patient with history of trauma or as a result of anticoagulation. This can then progress on to a subacute phase. Isodense SDH is a separate radiological entity where the blood products within a SDH have a CT density similar to adjacent brain. Chronic SDH is typically seen in the elderly patient, who may or may not have a clear history of head injury. As the brain atrophies, the subdural space enlarges (between the dura and arachnoid matter). A chronic SDH occurs when the bridging cortical veins within the subdural space are disrupted. Fresh bleeding within an existing chronic SHD is called acute upon chronic SDH.

Key facts
- Unenhanced CT is the first-line imaging investigation
- The haemorrhage may be acute, subacute, isodense or chronic depending on the attenuation of the haemorrhage
- It is important to distinguish an EDH from SDH (**Table 8.1**)

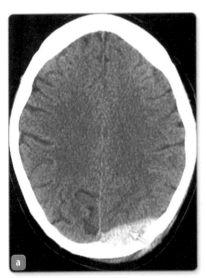

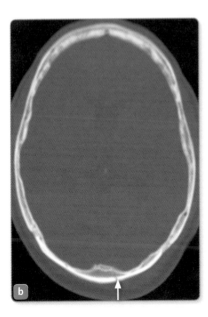

Figure 8.12 (a) CT scan of an acute left occipital extradural haemorrhage (arrow). (b) CT scan of underlying skull fracture (arrow) causing an acute extradural haemorrhage.

Feature	EDH	SDH
Location	Inner table of skull and dura	Between dura and arachnoid matter
Shape	Extra-axial and biconvex lens shape with underlying skull fracture (**Figure 8.12a** and **8.12b**)	Acute: concave-convex (hyperdense) Chronic: biconvex (hypodense)
Suture lines	Doesn't cross	Crosses
Tentorium	Can cross	Doesn't cross
Onset	Acute	Acute/chronic or acute on chronic (**Figure 8.13-8.16b**)

Table 8.1 A comparison of radiological signs in extradural (EDH) and subdural haematomas (SDH).

Radiographic findings

CT On an unenhanced CT scan, acute SDH has a concavo–convex shape and is hyperdense (**Figure 8.13**). In the subacute phase, a layering of blood is seen as a hyperdense component of blood cells and a low attenuation component of plasma (**Figure 8.14**). This then leads to the isodense phase of SDH where the blood products within the collection have a similar CT density to the adjacent brain (**Figure 8.15**). The only imaging clue to this condition will be mass effect and possible midline shift. Chronic SDH has a biconvex configuration and is hypodense relative to brain (**Figure 8.16a**). Hyperdense areas within a hypodense chronic SDH represent acute upon chronic SDH (**Figure 8.16b**).

Key signs
- Acute SDH is extra axial and concavo–convex in shape
- Subacute SDH shows a layering effect
- Isodense SDH is difficult to localise and mass effect/midline shift is a clue
- Chronic SDH is biconvex and hypodense

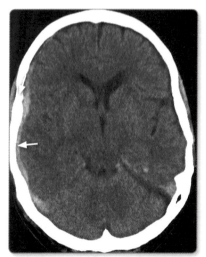

Figure 8.13 CT scan of an acute right subdural haemorrhage (arrows).

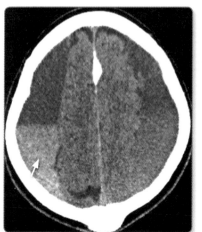

Figure 8.14 CT scan of bilateral subacute subdural haemorrhages. The right subdural haemorrhage demonstrates layering of blood (arrow).

- Acute upon chronic SDH shows hyperdense fresh blood within a hypodense chronic collection

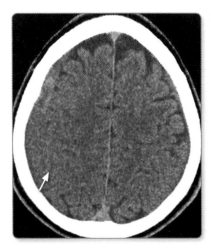

Figure 8.15 CT scan of an isodense subdural haemorrhage (arrow).

Management

When SDH is demonstrated on CT, a neurosurgical referral should be made, although surgical management of the patient will be guided by the degree of mass effect and underlying cause for haemorrhage. In theory, small SDH are treated conservatively and the patient will need follow-up CT to ensure that the haemorrhage has not increased in size.

8.5 Subarachnoid haemorrhage

SAH is haemorrhage into the subarachnoid space (between the arachnoid and pia mater). The incidence of SAH has been recorded as 10.5 per 100,000 person-years. The classic presentation is of a patient presenting acutely with 'the worst headache ever', mostly occipital and neck stiffness. It can mimic acute meningitis.

SAH can occur spontaneously or secondary to trauma. Ruptured aneurysm in the Circle of Willis is accountable for the majority of primary SAH. Complications include vasospasm leading to infarction, hydrocephalus and rebleeding. Rebleeding is associated with a mortality rate of over 40%.

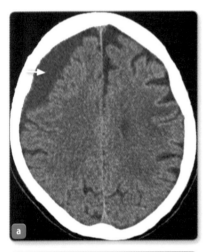

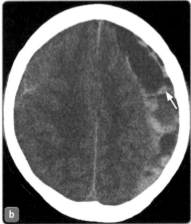

Figure 8.16 (a) CT scan of a chronic right subdural haemorrhage. Note how the chronic haemorrhage is now low attenuation in comparison to the acute haemorrhage. (b) CT scan of an acute on chronic left subdural haemorrhage.

Key facts

- Unenhanced CT is the first-line imaging investigation; however, a negative CT does not exclude a SAH
- If SAH is still suspected, a lumbar puncture is warranted for CSF analysis

Radiographic findings

CT On an unenhanced CT, SAH is seen as hyperdensity in the basal cisterns, sulci and within ventricles (**Figure 8.17a**). This can result in hydrocephalus. The earliest sign of hydrocephalus will be prominence of the temporal horns of the lateral ventricles (**Figure 8.17b**). Remember, a normal scan does not exclude a SAH.

Key signs
- Normal scan
- High attenuation in basal cisterns, sulci and ventricles
- Hydrocephalus

Management
Urgent neurosurgical referral should be made if CT is positive. The patient will then undergo a CT angiogram (CTA) or a catheter cerebral angiogram to locate a possible underlying aneurysm. Coiling of an aneurysm is a radiological procedure but sometimes patients need surgical management of the aneurysm.

If CT is normal, the patient will need a lumbar puncture and CSF analysis for red blood cells and xanthochromia. This will confirm the diagnosis of SAH.

8.6 Carotid/vertebral artery dissection

Dissection refers to haemorrhage within the vessel wall as a result of an intimal tear. This may be subintimal or subadventitial, resulting in luminal narrowing, vessel occlusion or pseudoaneurysm formation in the latter. Carotid or vertebral dissection is a leading cause of stroke in younger patients, and accounts for 5–20% of strokes. Internal carotid or vertebral artery dissection can occur secondary to trauma.

Patients may present with headache or neck pain. Internal carotid artery dissection may present with retro-orbital pain and acute Horner's syndrome. Pain precedes neurological signs, with patients presenting with transient ischaemic attacks (TIA) or strokes from 24 hours up to 10 days after the event. These

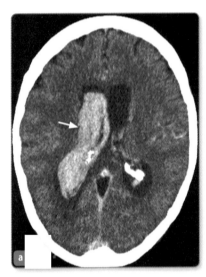

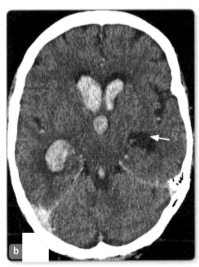

Figure 8.17 (a) CT of an acute subarachnoid haemorrhage, with blood within the ventricles (arrows). (b) CT demonstrating the prominent temporal horns (arrow) in a young patient with SAH, indicating hydrocephalus.

neurological complications result from luminal compromise and embolism.

Key facts
- Internal carotid dissection commonly occurs in the cervical segment just beyond the carotid bifurcation and, if present at C2/C3 level, will present clinically as acute Horner's syndrome
- Vertebral artery dissections commonly occur at C1/C2 level
- Pain and neurological signs should make you consider internal carotid or vertebral artery dissection

Radiographic findings

CTA CTA of the intra- and extracranial vessels is the imaging modality of choice when the patient presents acutely. This will allow adequate assessment for dissection as well as associated complications including stroke. The lumen of the dissected segment of the artery will be narrowed due to the intramural haematoma (**Figure 8.18a**). Other findings include a false lumen with dissection flap, total vessel occlusion and proximal/distal dilatation.

MRI Magnetic resonance imaging (MRI) is another imaging modality used to demonstrate intramural haematoma in a patient with dissection. On T1 weighted fat saturation imaging (axial), the intramural haematoma will be seen as high signal within the vessel wall, confirming the diagnosis (**Figure 8.18b**).

Key signs
- Luminal narrowing of the vessel at site of dissection
- Intramural haematoma on MRI
- Vessel occlusion
- Stroke

Management
The aim of management is to prevent neurological injury as a result of embolic stroke. Medical management includes antiplatelets and anticoagulation.

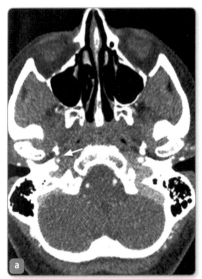

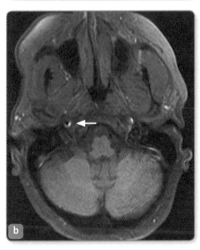

Figure 8.18 (a) CT angiogram showing narrowing of the lumen of the right internal carotid artery (arrow) in comparison to the left. (b) MR T1 fat-saturated image illustrating dissection of the right internal carotid artery (arrow).

8.7 Stroke

Stroke is characterised by rapidly developing focal neurological deficits lasting more than 24 hours. In developed countries, stroke is the third most common cause of death. Transient ischaemic attack is a term used when the symptoms and signs resolve within 48 hours. These patients require assessment and optimisation of risk factors to prevent a stroke.

> ### Clinical insight
>
> When taking a clinical history, remember to elicit risk factors for stroke/TIA, including:
>
> - Age
> - Hypertension
> - Diabetes
> - Cardiovascular disease
> - Atrial fibrillation
> - Hypercholesterolaemia
> - Smoking
> - Family history

Approximately 80% of acute strokes are due to arterial disease resulting in infarction of the brain. The most common cause of stroke is atherosclerosis of the Circle of Willis. Other causes include embolic infarction, secondary to conditions like atrial fibrillation and carotid artery stenosis. Stroke can also occur secondary to intracerebral or subarachnoid haemorrhage.

Key facts

- The patient can present with focal neurological deficit depending on the arterial territory involved
- Haemorrhagic transformation occurs due to blood extravasating into the infarcted brain and is seen mostly in embolic stroke

Radiographic findings

CT Unenhanced CT scan is the first line of investigation. An area of acute infarction will be of low attenuation (**Figure 8.19a**). This is due to cytotoxic oedema as a result of poor perfusion of the affected part of the brain and resultant cell death. This will lead to loss of gray–white matter differentiation, effacement of sulci and, if large, mass effect. The CT scan can be normal if performed less than 6 hours from the onset of symptoms and signs. However, there may be subtle clues to hyperacute infarction, which include the 'hyperdense MCA sign' (**Figure 8.19b**). The proximal segment of the middle cerebral artery (MCA) will

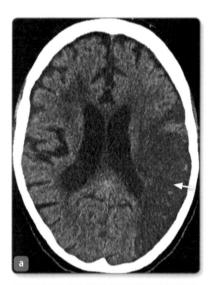

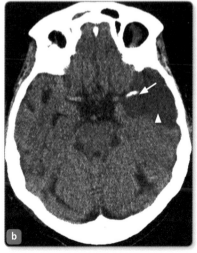

Figure 8.19 (a) CT scan of an infarction in the left middle cerebral artery territory (arrow). (b) CT scan demonstrating the 'hyperdense middle cerebral artery (MCA) sign'. There is high attenuation in the left MCA in keeping with thrombus (arrow) which has resulted in infarction (arrowhead).

show high attenuation. Other subtle signs include effacement of the Sylvian fissure, also called the 'insular ribbon sign', loss of gray–white differentiation and loss of definition of basal ganglia structures.

The area of brain affected will depend on the arterial territory involved. For example, an occipital lobe infarction (**Figure 8.20**) will be due to a posterior cerebral artery territory infarction.

MRI MRI is the modality of choice in a patient suspected of having had a TIA. On diffusion-weighted images, an acute infarction will demonstrate restricted diffusion and appear bright (**Figure 8.21**). MR angiography is also performed to visualise the state of the intracranial arterial circulation.

Key signs

- Low attenuation extending to cortex
- Loss of gray–white matter differentiation
- Hyperdense MCA sign
- Mass effect and midline shift

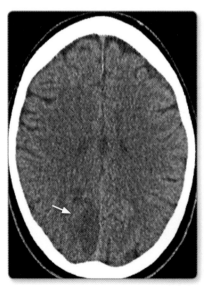

Figure 8.20 CT scan demonstrating an acute right posterior cerebral artery infarct in the occipital lobe.

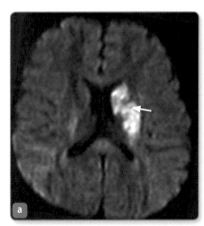

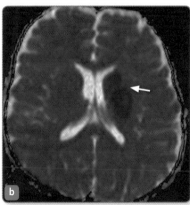

Figure 8.21 (a) MR diffusion-weighted image showing restricted diffusion in acute left basal ganglia infarction (arrow). (b) MR apparent diffusion coefficient map showing low signal in the corresponding area to Figure 8.12 (arrow), confirming restricted diffusion and acute infarction.

Management

The aim of management is to reduce mortality, impairment, disability and secondary complications. This is achieved by a multidisciplinary team approach to patient management, involving stroke physicians, nurses, physiotherapists, speech and language therapists, and occupational therapists. In many centres, patients may undergo thrombolysis (either intravenous or intra-arterial) in acute stroke.

8.8 Cerebral venous thrombosis

Cerebral venous thrombosis (CVT) may affect both cerebral veins and dural venous sinuses. It is often a difficult diagnosis as its presentation is non-specific, with symptoms including headache and visual disturbances. There are many predisposing factors which include hypercoagulable states, infection, malignancy, trauma and iatrogenic (e.g. indwelling catheters).

Key facts
- Cerebral venous thrombosis often presents as infarction not confined to the vascular territory
- Haemorrhagic infarction not confined to a vascular territory distribution is a pointer to the diagnosis of venous infarction
- In the acute setting, CT venogram is the investigation of choice

Radiographic findings

CT On unenhanced CT scan, signs of CVT include thrombus within a dural sinus, infarctions in a non-arterial distribution and bilateral involvement (**Figure 8.22**). A normal CT venogram will demonstrate good opacification of the venous sinuses with contrast. In venous thrombosis, there will be filling defects within the affected cerebral veins/dural sinuses.

MRI On T1 weighted sequences, the thrombosed vessels will demonstrate lack of flow void. Slow flow within the vessel will appear hyperintense. A normal MR venogram will demonstrate high signal in the veins and sinuses. In the presence of a thrombosis there will be reduced flow in these vessels resulting in loss of the normal signal from the vessel (**Figure 8.23**).

Key signs
- CT venogram demonstrates a filling defect at the site of thrombosis
- Infarction in non-arterial distribution
- T1 MRI sequence shows absence of flow voids in the affected vessel(s) and high signal
- MR venogram demonstrates reduced or no flow in affected veins/sinuses

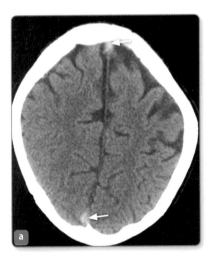

Figure 8.22 (a) CT scans demonstrating high attenuation in the superior sagittal venous sinus, in keeping with thrombosis (arrows). (b) CT scan of venous infarction and associated haemorrhage in the right parietal lobe (arrow), due to venous sinus infarction.

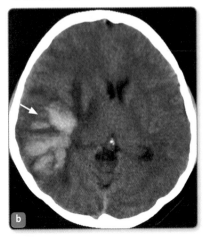

Management

Patients recovering from cerebral vein/dural sinus thrombosis are at risk of recurrent thrombosis. It is important to establish underlying risk factors for thrombosis. Anticoagulation is prescribed for 3–6 months, following the first episode.

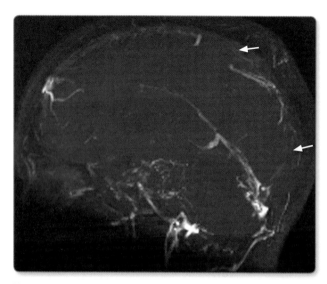

Figure 8.23 A time-of-flight MR venogram showing absence of opacification of the superior sagittal sinus (arrows), in keeping with venous sinus thrombosis.

8.9 Space-occupying lesions

Common space-occupying lesions include primary malignancies, metastasis and abscess. The diagnosis depends upon clinical history, physical examination and radiological characteristics of the mass. The patient can present acutely with headaches and signs of raised intracranial pressure. This is a neurological emergency and urgent investigation is required.

Key facts

- Differentiating abscess from malignancy radiologically can be very difficult. Clinical history and examination are crucial to help differentiate between the two. Age of patient, location of lesion and characteristics can help provide a differential diagnosis for space-occupying lesions
- A patient presenting with headaches, fever, neck stiffness, photophobia and raised inflammatory markers is likely to have an intracranial infection and abscess formation

- It is important to provide a history of known malignancy on the request card

Radiographic findings

CT CT scan before and after contrast is the initial investigation of choice. It is important to evaluate the pressure effects of the mass lesion (**Figure 8.24**). These include mass effect, midline shift and herniation. There can be associated with vasogenic oedema.

MRI Performing MRI before and after contrast can help further characterise space-occupying lesions. The signal characteristics and location of the space-occupying lesion, i.e. intra- or extra-axial, can help provide an appropriate differential diagnosis. Diffusion-weighted imaging can help differentiate an abscess from malignancy.

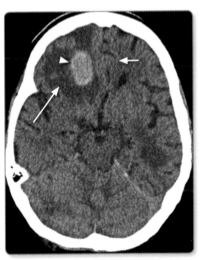

Figure 8.24 CT scan with contrast showing a mass lesion (arrowhead) and surrounding vasogenic oedema (long arrow). There is associated mass effect and subfalcine herniation (arrow).

Key signs

- Mass lesion
- Intra- or extra-axial in location
- Necrosis, haemorrhage, cystic component, calcification
- Enhancement after contrast administration can vary
- Vasogenic oedema with mass effect and midline shift

Management

Further management will depend on the nature of the mass lesion. This may require further imaging like MRI and neuro-surgical input.

Musculoskeletal system

9.1 Key radiological anatomy

Cervical spine

The cervical spine consists of seven cervical vertebrae. Cervical spine injuries can initially be assessed by plain radiograph. A lateral radiograph, odontoid view and anteroposterior (AP) view radiograph are usually requested.

Lateral view

In assessing lateral view radiographs of the cervical spine (**Figure 9.1**):

- Adequacy of the radiograph is assessed, for which the C7/T1 junction Ⓐ must be seen

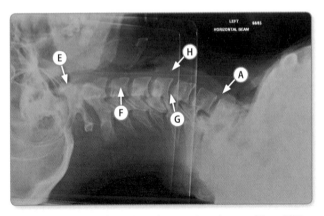

Figure 9.1 Lateral cervical-spine X-ray demonstrating adequacy of X-ray: C7/T1 junction Ⓐ, atlanto-axial distance Ⓔ, uniform vertebral body Ⓕ, intervertebral disc size and shape Ⓖ, and normal prevertebral soft tissues Ⓗ.

- Vertebral alignment is evaluated by tracing three lines and ensuring they are continuous with no disruptions. Trace the anterior margins of the vertebral bodies (**line** Ⓑ, the posterior margins of the vertebral bodies (**line** Ⓒ), and the spinous processes bases (**line** Ⓓ) (**Figure 9.2**)
- Assess the atlanto-axial distance, which should be <3 mm in adults Ⓔ
- Vertebral body shape and heights should be uniform and equal throughout the spine Ⓕ
- Intervertebral disc heights should be equal Ⓖ
- Prevertebral soft tissue – the normal width of the soft tissue at C1–4 level should be ≤7 mm and at C5–7 level it should be ≤22 mm Ⓗ

Odontoid view

Odontoid view radiographs of the cervical spine (**Figure 9.3**) demonstrate the C1 and C2 articulation; the lateral margins of C1 should align with those of C2 Ⓘ and there should be an equal distance between the odontoid peg and the lateral mass of C2 on either side Ⓙ.

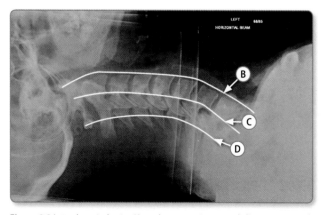

Figure 9.2 Lateral cervical-spine X-ray demonstrating normal alignment: normal anterior vertebral alignment (line Ⓑ), posterior vertebral alignment (line Ⓒ) and alignment of the spinous processes (line Ⓓ).

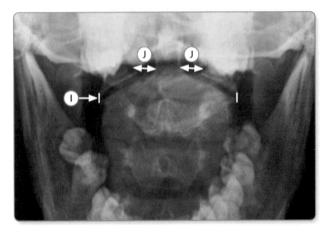

Figure 9.3 Odontoid view X-ray demonstrating normal alignment of the lateral masses of C1 and C2 (I) and distance between the odontoid peg and lateral masses of C1 (J).

AP view

The AP view of the C spine (**Figure 9.4**) demonstrates the uncovertebral joints (K) and spinous process alignment (L), which should be in line, and there should be an equal distance between the spinous process tips (M)

Thoracic spine

The thoracic spine is made up of 12 load-bearing vertebrae that articulate with the rib cage. Thoracic spine injuries can be assessed on radiographs as well as CT. Lateral and AP radiographs are standard views.

Lateral view

In assessing lateral view radiographs of the thoracic spine (**Figure 9.5**):

- Vertebral alignment is assessed by tracing two lines and ensuring they are continuous with no disruptions. Trace the anterior margins of the vertebral bodies (**line** (N)) and the posterior margins of the vertebral bodies (**line** (O))

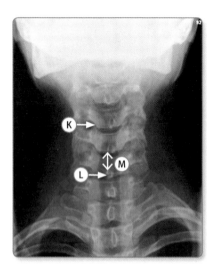

Figure 9.4 An anteroposterior cervical-spine X-ray demonstrating the uncovertebral joints (K), spinous processes (L), and distance between the spinous processes (M).

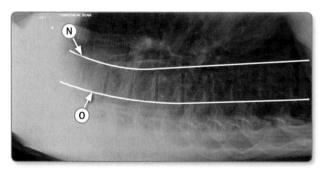

Figure 9.5 Lateral thoracic spine X-ray demonstrating normal alignment: normal anterior vertebral alignment (line (N)) and posterior vertebral alignment (line (O)).

- Evaluate the vertebral body shape and heights; the anterior vertebral height is 2–3 mm less than the posterior height, producing a mild kyphosis
- Intervertebral disc heights should be equal

AP view

In assessing AP view radiographs of the thoracic spine (**Figure 9.6**):

- Vertebral body shape, heights and pedicles ⓟ should be assessed. The AP diameter of the vertebral bodies gradually increases from T1 to T12, and the transverse diameter of the vertebral bodies gradually increases from T3 to T12
- The left paraspinal line is produced by the interface between the lung and paravertebral soft tissues and is adjacent to the vertebral bodies (**line** ⓠ)

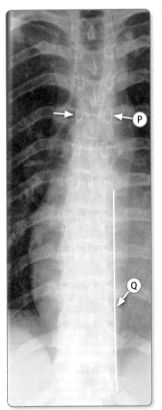

Figure 9.6 An anteroposterior thoracic spine X-ray demonstrating the pedicles ⓟ and the left paraspinal line (line ⓠ).

Lumbar spine

The lumbar spine is made up of five load-bearing vertebrae. Lumbar spine injuries can be assessed on radiographs as well as CT. A lateral and an AP radiograph are required.

Lateral view

In assessing lateral view radiographs of the lumbar spine (**Figure 9.7**):

- Vertebral alignment is assessed by tracing two lines and ensuring they are continuous with no disruptions. Trace the anterior margins of the vertebral bodies (**line Ⓡ**) and the posterior margins of the vertebral bodies (**line Ⓢ**)
- Vertebral body shape and heights should be uniform and equal, both anteriorly and posteriorly
- Intervertebral disc heights should also be equal

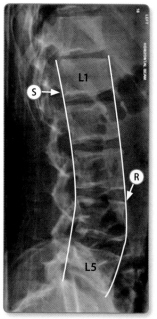

Figure 9.7 Lateral lumbar spine X-ray demonstrating normal alignment: normal anterior vertebral alignment (line Ⓡ) and posterior vertebral alignment (line Ⓢ).

AP view

In assessing AP view radiographs of the lumbar spine (**Figure 9.8**); assess vertebral body shape, heights, pedicles and transverse processes (T).

Spinal stability

Spinal stability has been described in different ways. However, the aim is to identify whether the injury is stable or unstable. The 'three column spine theory' helps in the assessment of the spine and to determine its stability (**Figure 9.9**):

- **Anterior column** (U): this consists of the ALL (anterior longitudinal ligament), the anterior two-thirds of the vertebral body and the anterior part of the annulus fibrosus
- **Middle column** (V): this consists of the PLL (posterior longitudinal ligament), the posterior third of the vertebral body and the posterior part of the annulus fibrosus

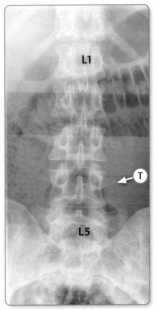

Figure 9.8 An anteroposterior lumbar spine X-ray demonstrating the transverse processes (T).

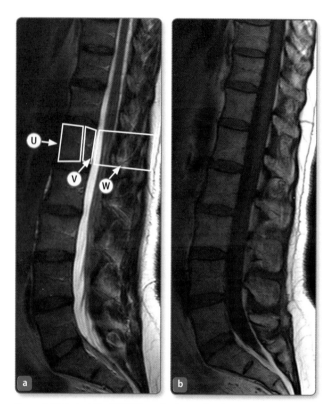

Figure 9.9 Spinal stability. (a) MR T2-weighted sagittal lumbar spine image demonstrating three column spinal stability: anterior column Ⓤ, middle column Ⓥ and posterior column Ⓦ. (b) MR sagittal lumbar spine image demonstrating normal vertebral alignment.

- **Posterior column** Ⓦ: this consists of the pedicles, laminae, facets, transverse processes, spinous processes and the posterior ligaments

Spinal injuries involving only the vertebral body *or* the posterior elements are stable. These injuries involve only one column. Spinal injuries involving *both* vertebral body *and* posterior elements are unstable. These injuries involve more than one of the spinal columns.

9.2 Cervical spine injuries

Cervical spine injuries account for two-thirds of spinal cord injuries, with the lower cervical spine the most common site of injury. Many factors are associated with a higher risk of cervical spine injury. These include a decreased Glasgow Coma Scale (GCS) score, loss of consciousness, neck tenderness, neurological deficit and a significant force of injury (e.g. high-speed road traffic collision (RTC)).

Cervical spine injuries can be classified according to the mechanism of injury. This includes hyperflexion, hyperextension, flexion–rotation, vertical compression and lateral flexion injuries. (**Table 9.1**).

> **Clinical insight**
>
> There is a high risk of associated injury in patients with cervical spine injuries. Once a primary survey has been completed, a thorough secondary survey should be performed to elicit any further injuries.

Key facts

- Hyperflexion injuries are the most common injury of the cervical spine
- Plain radiographs may be completely normal in cervical spine injuries
- It is important to visualise the C7/T1 junction as fractures may be missed at this site (**Figure 9.10**)
- Care needs to be taken in managing patients with unstable cervical spine injuries to prevent further spinal cord injury

Radiographic findings

Plain radiograph and CT Direct signs of fracture on the lateral radiograph include loss of normal alignment, change in shape and size of vertebral body, increase in atlanto-axial distance and widening of the prevertebral soft tissue shadow. On the AP view, uncovertebral dislocation and unilateral facet joint dislocation can be assessed. The odontoid view may demonstrate disruption of the normal alignment of the lateral masses and an odontoid fracture (**Figure 9.11**). This finding is better demonstrated on CT reconstructed in both sagittal and coronal planes (**Figure 9.12**).

Mechanism of injury	Injury sustained	Stability
Hyperflexion	Odontoid fracture (**Figures 9.10–9.12**)	Unstable
Hyperflexion	Flexion teardrop fracture resulting in avulsion of the anteroinferior corner of the vertebral body by the ALL. This injury is associated with ligamentous injuries and spinal cord injury (**Figures 9.13** and **9.14**)	Unstable
Hyperflexion	Bilateral facet dislocation with interlocking of the facet joints. This injury results in anterolisthesis of the involved vertebrae, but no rotational deformity (**Figures 9.14**)	Unstable
Hyperflexion	Spinous process fracture as a result of a sudden load onto a flexed cervical spine. These injuries commonly involve C6/C7 or T1 spinous processes	Stable
Hyperextension	Bilateral pars fracture of C2 (hangman's fracture). This fracture is associated with dislocation of C2 on C3 (**Figure 9.15**)	Unstable
Flexion–rotation	Unilateral facet dislocation resulting in rotation of the spinous processes and uncovertebral joints on AP view	Stable
Vertical compression	Burst fracture of C1 (Jefferson fracture). This injury results in disruption of the anterior and posterior arches of C1	Unstable

Table 9.1 Types of unstable and stable cervical spine injuries.

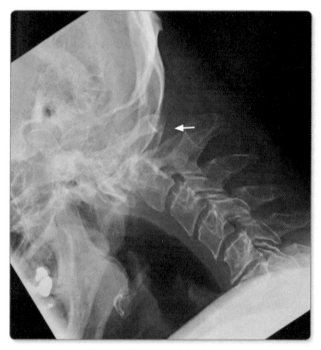

Figure 9.10 An inadequate lateral cervical-spine X-ray which does not demonstrate the C7/T1 junction. There is disruption of the normal alignment of the vertebral bodies and spinous processes at C1 and C2 (arrow).

MRI Magnetic resonance imaging (MRI) will help assess associated spinal cord and ligamentous injuries. High signal within the cord at the level of injury on T2 weighted imaging indicates a cord injury. An associated intramedullary haematoma will have a well-defined area of low signal surrounding the abnormal high T2 signal.

Key signs
- Disruption to normal alignment
- Widening of the interspinous distance
- Widening of the facet joints

- Widening of prevertebral soft tissue shadow
- Normal radiograph
- Spinal cord injury on MRI

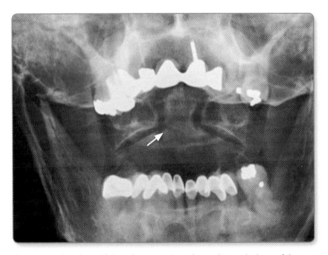

Figure 9.11 An odontoid view demonstrating a lucent line at the base of the odontoid peg (arrow) in keeping with a fracture.

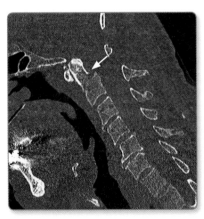

Figure 9.12 Sagittal CT reconstruction demonstrating odontoid fracture (arrow).

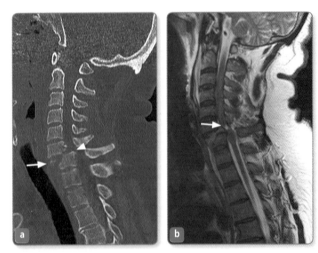

Figure 9.13 Flexion teardrop fracture. (a) Sagittal CT reconstruction demonstrating a flexion teardrop fracture. There is avulsion of the anterior corner of the C7 vertebral body (arrow) and dislocation of C6 on C7 (arrowhead). (b) Sagittal MR T2-weighted image demonstrating spinal cord transection (arrow) as a result of flexion teardrop fracture.

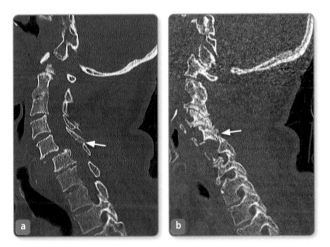

Figure 9.14 Sagittal CT reconstructions demonstrating bilateral facet joint dislocation (arrows) with dislocation of C5 on C6.

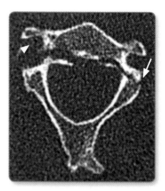

Figure 9.15 Axial CT demonstrating bilateral pars fractures of C2 vertebra (arrow). On the right the fracture extends into the right transverse foramen (arrowhead).

Management

Patients suspected of sustaining a cervical spine injury should have spinal immobilisation in place. Once a cervical spine injury has been diagnosed, a referral to the spinal surgeons should be made, who will decide on further management.

9.3 Thoracic spine injuries

Thoracic spine injuries result from compression, impaction and shearing forces. Upper thoracic spine fractures (T1–T10) are relatively stable due to the thoracic cage and strong costovertebral ligaments.

The majority of thoracic spine injuries commonly occur at the thoracolumbar junction (T11–L2) as a result of transition from a relatively immobile to a mobile spine.

Key facts

- Simple wedge or compression fractures occur from compressive forces transmitted through the longitudinal axis of the spine, resulting in anterior wedging of the vertebral body
- Direct impact (e.g. a fall onto the back) results in fractures of the vertebral bodies, posterior elements and injuries to the costovertebral joints

- Fracture/dislocation injuries occur as a result of shearing forces at the thoracolumbar junction. This very unstable fracture results in injury to all three spinal columns secondary to a horizontal impacting force

Radiographic findings

Plain radiograph and CT Direct signs of thoracic spine injury include disruption of normal alignment and change in shape/size of the vertebral bodies on the lateral view (**Figure 9.16a**). An AP view will demonstrate widening of the left paraspinal line, loss of height of the vertebral body and obscuration of pedicles (**Figure 9.16b**). These findings can be better appreciated on CT reconstructed in the coronal and sagittal planes.

Key signs
- Disruption to normal alignment
- Loss of height of vertebral body
- 'Winking owl' sign – obscured pedicle
- Disruption of more than one spinal column

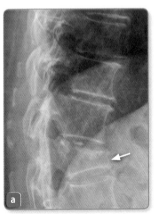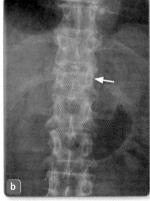

Figure 9.16 Wedge fractures of T12 vertebra. (a) Lateral thoracic spine X-ray demonstrating a wedge fracture of T12 with loss of vertebral height (arrow). (b) An anteroposterior thoracic spine X-ray demonstrating a wedge fracture of T12 (arrow). There is loss of height of the vertebral body.

Management

Further management of the patient will depend on the severity and stability of the injury sustained. Referral to spinal surgeons should be made.

9.4 Lumbar spine injuries

Lumbar spine injuries commonly occur at the thoracolumbar junction (T11–L2). Fractures are classed as stable or unstable depending on the spinal columns disrupted.

Key facts

- Simple wedge fractures are the most common lumbar spine injury and involve the superior end plate
- Burst fractures can occur in thoracolumbar injuries, resulting in retropulsion of the superoposterior margin of the

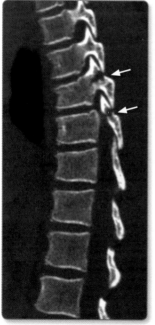

Figure 9.17 Sagittal CT reconstruction demonstrating a chance-type injury, with horizontal fractures through the posterior elements of the lower thoracic spine (arrow).

vertebral body into the spinal canal. This can result in compression of the spinal cord, conus medullaris or cauda equina

- Seatbelt injury (i.e. 'chance fractures', **Figure 9.17**): an example of these unstable injuries is a horizontal fracture through the vertebral body into the posterior elements (**Figure 9.18**). Seatbelt injuries commonly occur at the L2 or L3 vertebral levels as a result of a shearing flexion/distraction injury

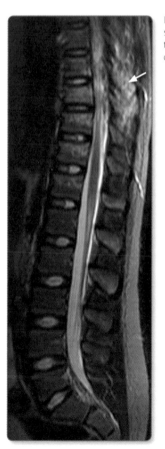

Figure 9.18 Sagittal MR T2-weighted scan demonstrating high signal within the spinous ligaments as a result of chance-type injury (arrow).

- Isolated transverse process fractures can result from direct local injury or avulsion of the psoas muscle

Radiographic findings

Plain radiograph Direct signs of lumbar spine injury include disruption of normal alignment, change in shape/size of the vertebral bodies, and retropulsion of a fracture fragment into the spinal canal on the lateral view (**Figure 9.19a**). The AP view may demonstrate loss of height of the vertebral body and obscuration of pedicles (**Figure 9.19b**). These findings are well-demonstrated on CT reconstructed in the coronal and sagittal planes (**Figure 9.20a**).

MRI MRI images will demonstrate retropulsion of a fracture fragment into the spinal canal (**Figure 9.20b**). Associated spinal cord/conus medullaris or cauda equina injuries can be diagnosed on MRI. Sagittal MR images will demonstrate abnormal high T2 signal within the spinal cord as well as posterior ligamentous injuries.

Key signs
- Disruption to normal alignment
- Loss of height of vertebral body
- 'Winking owl' sign – obscured pedicle
- Disruption of more than one spinal column with retropulsion of a fracture fragment into spinal canal

Management
Further management of the patient will depend on the severity and stability of the injury sustained. Referral to spinal surgeons should be made.

9.5 Cauda equina compression

Cauda equina compression is an emergency that requires prompt diagnosis and management. Patients present with 'red flag' symptoms and signs that compose the cauda equina syndrome. These include radicular pain (back, buttocks, perineum and legs), decreased sensation and weakness in the lumbar

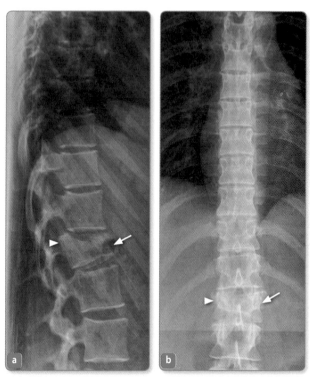

Figure 9.19 Wedge fractures of L1. (a) Lateral spine X-ray demonstrating a wedge fracture of L1 (arrow). There is a loss of height of the vertebral body with retropulsion of the posterior vertebral body into the spinal canal (arrowhead). (b) Anteroposterior spine X-ray demonstrating a wedge fracture of L1 (arrow). There is a loss of height of the vertebral body and loss of the right pedicle (arrowhead).

and sacral dermatomes and myotomes, decreased ankle reflexes, disturbed sphincter function, overflow/incontinence, decreased sphincter tone and impotence. If a diagnosis of cauda equina

Clinical insight

In a patient presenting with low back pain it is vital to elicit symptoms of cauda equina syndrome and conduct a full neurological examination of the lower limbs as well as a rectal examination to elicit anal tone and perianal paraesthesia.

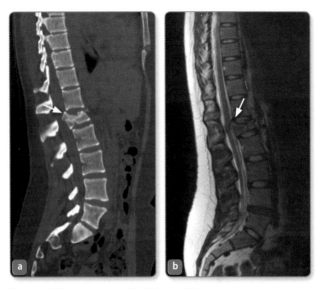

Figure 9.20 Wedge fractures of L1. (a) Sagittal CT reconstruction demonstrating L1 wedge fracture with retropulsion into the spinal canal (arrow). (b) Sagittal MR T2-weighted scan demonstrating L1 wedge fracture with retropulsed fragment abutting the spinal cord (arrow).

compression is missed, it can lead to devastating consequences for the patient.

Key facts
- Cauda equina compression results from a compressive lesion in the lower lumbar spinal canal
- It occurs commonly as a result of an intervertebral disc prolapse. Other causes include masses and degenerative disease resulting in spinal stenosis
- The imaging modality of choice is MRI

Radiographic findings

MRI MRI is the imaging modality of choice to diagnose cauda equina (**Figure 9.21**).

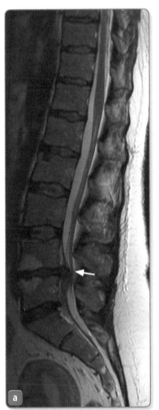

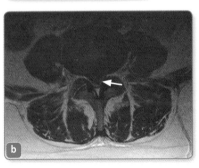

Figure 9.21 Cauda equina compression. (a) Sagittal MR T2-weighted scan demonstrating a large L4/L5 disc prolapsed and compressing the cauda equina (arrow). (b) Axial MR T2-weighted scan demonstrating a large L4/L5 disc prolapsed and compressing the cauda equina (arrow).

Key signs
- Displaced prolapsed disc or mass in spinal canal
- Narrowing of the spinal canal and compression of the cauda equina
- Spinal stenosis as a result of degenerative disease (facet joint osteoarthrtis and ligamentum hypertrophy)

Management
Urgent referral needs to be made to spinal surgeons for emergency decompression of the cauda equina compression.

9.6 Spondylodiscitis

Spondylodiscitis is infection within the spine due to haematogenous spread of bacteria that invades the vertebral body infecting the relatively avascular intervertebral disc. Other causes for discitis include invasive procedures (e.g. surgery, myelography). Patients will present with back pain, pyrexia and raised inflammatory markers.

Key facts
- A common pathogen for pyogenic discitis is *Staphylococcus aureus*
- Non-pyogenic discitis pathogens include tuberculosis (TB)
- Discitis commonly occurs at the L3/L4 or L4/L5 levels
- Discitis is the most common paediatric spine problem

Radiographic findings

Plain radiograph In the early stages, plain radiograph may be normal. Radiograph signs of discitis include disc space narrowing, loss of definition of the end plates and paravertebral swelling.

MRI This is the modality of choice and is very sensitive in detecting early disease. On T1 weighted images, a decrease in fatty marrow signal in two contiguous vertebrae is seen (**Figure 9.22a**). In early disease, the disc height may be preserved; however, there may be high T2 signal within it (**Figure 9.22b**). As the disease

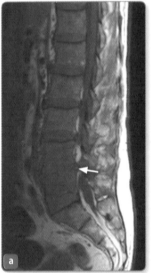

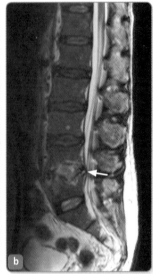

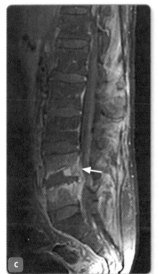

Figure 9.22 Spondylodiscitis.
(a) Sagittal MR T1-weighted scan
demonstrating abnormal signal return
from L4 and L5 vertebral bodies
(arrow). (b) Sagittal MR T2-weighted
scan demonstrating abnormal signal
return from the L4/L5 intervertebral
disc and the end plates of the vertebral
bodies (arrow). (c) Sagittal MR T1W
post contrast scan demonstrating
abnormal enhancement of L4 and
L5 vertebral bodies in keeping with
infection (arrow).

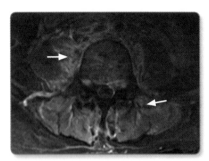

Figure 9.23 Axial MR
T1-weighted post-contrast
scan demonstrating
discitis with abnormal
enhancement of the
paraspinal and posterior
vertebral soft tissues
(arrows).

progresses, the disc height will be reduced with increasing T2
signal. Post contrast imaging will reveal abnormal enhancement
of the intervertebral disc and associated paravertebral soft tissue
swelling (**Figures 9.22c** and **9.23**). As infected material from the
disc protrudes into the spinal canal, an epidural abscess may
form, indenting the anterior thecal sac.

Key signs
- Disc space narrowing
- Irregularity of the vertebral end plates
- Paravertebral soft tissue swelling
- Spinal epidural abscess

Management
Referral to spinal surgeons should be made for emergency
decompression.

Paediatric emergency imaging

10.1 Upper gastrointestinal (GI) tract disorders

Duodenal atresia

Duodenal atresia presents in the neonate with bilious vomiting and is the most common cause of congenital duodenal obstruction. It results from a failure of canalisation of the duodenal lumen in utero. This condition can be detected on prenatal ultrasound (US) scan, especially if there is polyhydramnios.

Key facts

- Associated with Trisomy 21, other GI anomalies (e.g. oesophageal, biliary and small bowel atresia, malrotation, annular pancreas and Meckel's diverticulum) and congenital heart disease
- Commonly presents following the first feed
- Vomiting can lead to loss of fluids and electrolytes, and rapid deterioration

Radiographic findings

Plain radiograph The diagnosis of duodenal atresia is made on plain abdominal radiograph. The pathognomic finding is of the 'double bubble' sign, resulting from a distended stomach and proximal duodenum. Distal to this, bowel gas is absent (**Figure 10.1**).

Key signs

- 'Double bubble' sign
- Absence of small and large bowel gas

Management

Referral to paediatric surgeons is required for operative management of the duodenal atresia.

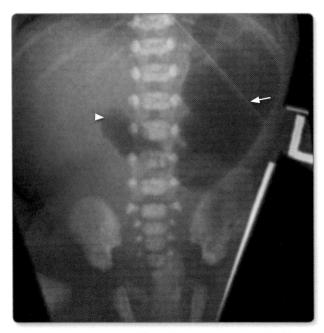

Figure 10.1 An anteroposterior abdominal X-ray demonstrating the double bubble sign. There is a nasogastric tube tip in the distended stomach (arrow). The proximal duodenum is distended (arrowhead), with no gas distally.

Malrotation

Malrotation results from aberrant embryology and abnormal fixation of the mesentery. The long mesenteric attachments to the duodenojejunal (DJ) flexure and the caecum, suspend the midgut and prevent volvulus. In malrotation, the mesenteric attachment is short, which predisposes to small bowel volvulus. If small bowel volvulus occurs, the superior mesenteric artery can obstruct, resulting in ischaemia and infarction of the midgut.

Key facts

- Malrotation commonly presents in neonates with bilious vomiting. However, it can present after 2 months of age with recurrent vomiting and distension

- Malrotation occurs in different degrees, from complete malrotation to incomplete rotation
- Associated with other congenital anomalies (e.g. Prune-belly syndrome)

Radiographic findings

Plain radiograph The stomach and proximal duodenum may be distended. However, the plain abdominal radiograph can be normal and does not exclude malrotation or volvulus.

Upper GI contrast study This is the modality used to establish the diagnosis of malrotation. A normal contrast study will demonstrate a normal DJ flexure to the left of the spine at the same level as the duodenal cap. Depending on the degree of malrotation, different findings will be seen on the contrast study. This can range from a mild degree of rotation with a low-lying DJ flexure to a more severe degree, where the DJ flexure cannot be identified.

Key signs

- Non-rotation – duodenum and entire small bowel lie on the right of the abdomen
- Malrotation – duodenum (**Figure 10.2a**) and jejunum to the right of the spine
- Malrotation – corkscrew duodenum and jejunum (**Figure 10.2b**)
- Malrotation – abnormal position of DJ flexure or not visualised

Management
Referral to paediatric surgeons is required for urgent operative management.

Hypertrophic pyloric stenosis
Hypertrophic pyloric stenosis is characterised by hypertrophy and hyperplasia of the circular muscles of the pylorus.

Key facts
- Pyloric stenosis commonly presents in the first 2 to 12 weeks of life with non-bilious projectile vomiting
- Associated with a positive family history and more common in males

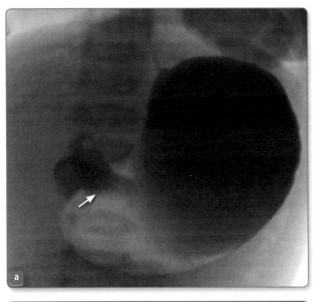

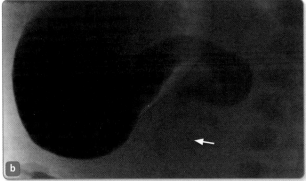

Figure 10.2 (a) Upper GI contrast study demonstrating a coiled distal duodenum with no visualisation of the duodenojejunal flexure (arrow). (b) Upper GI contrast study demonstrating corkscrew appearance of the jejunum (arrow).

- There may be an 'olive-shaped' mass palpable on clinical examination

Radiographic findings

US This is the modality of choice, demonstrating thickening of the pyloric muscle wall (>3 mm), an increased pyloric diameter (>15 mm) and an elongated pyloric channel (>16 mm) (**Figure 10.3**). Ultrasound may demonstrate a dilated fluid-filled antrum with the thickened pylorus indenting into it, the 'cervix sign'.

Key signs

- Elongated pyloric channel >16 mm (**Dimension 1, Figure 10.3**)

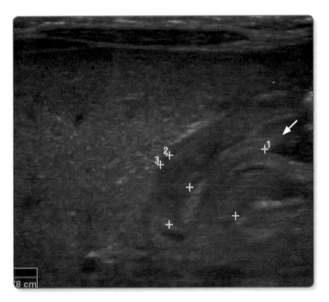

Figure 10.3 Abdominal US demonstrating pyloric thickening with elongation of the pylorus (dimension 1), increase in diameter of the pylorus (dimension 2) and thickening of the muscle wall (dimension 3). There is indentation of the thickened pylorus into the fluid-filled antrum (cervix sign) (arrow).

- Thickened pyloric diameter >15 mm (**Dimension 2, Figure 10.3**)
- Thickened pyloric muscle wall >3 mm (**Dimension 3, Figure 10.3**)
- Cervix sign

Management

Referral to paediatric surgeons is required for operative management.

10.2 Lower gastrointestinal tract disorders

Necrotising enterocolitis

Necrotising enterocolitis (NEC) is the most common surgical emergency in infants. Ischaemic bowel can result from hypoxia, perinatal stress, congenital heart disease and infection. NEC is a disorder of prematurity with the majority of cases occurring in neonates born at less than 36 weeks' gestation.

Key facts

- NEC commonly develops within the first 10 days of life
- Neonates can present with abdominal distension and bilious vomiting
- NEC usually occurs in the terminal ileum, followed by the caecum and right colon
- Delayed complications include bowel strictures and short gut syndrome from excessive bowel necrosis and resection

Radiographic findings

Plain radiograph Abdominal radiograph findings include distended bowel loops and bowel wall thickening. Bowel wall gas (pneumatosis intestinalis) is definitive for NEC, and commonly located in the right lower quadrant. Portal venous gas may also be seen on plain radiograph as branching lucencies projected over the liver, and is often transient. A bad prognostic sign is pneumoperitoneum, for which immediate surgery is required.

Key signs
- Dilatation of bowel
- Bowel wall thickening
- Pneumatosis intestinalis (**Figure 10.4**)
- Portal venous gas
- Pneumoperitoneum (**Figure 10.5**)

Management
NEC can be managed conservatively or surgically. Pneumo-peritoneum is an absolute indication for surgery and urgent referral to paediatric surgeons is required.

Intussusception
Intussusception occurs when a segment of bowel (the intus-susceptum) telescopes into a more distal segment of bowel (the intussuscipiens), resulting in bowel obstruction. Intussus-ception can be ileoileal or ileocolic. This is the most common abdominal emergency of early childhood, occurring from 6 months to 3 years of age.

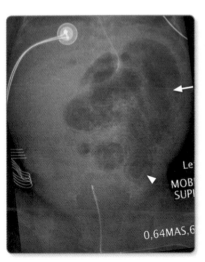

Figure 10.4 Abdominal X-ray demonstrating dilated bowel loops (arrow) and bowel wall gas (arrowhead).

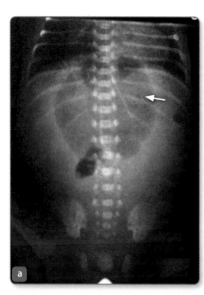

Figure 10.5 (a) Supine abdominal X-ray demonstrating pneumoperitoneum, 'the football sign' (arrow). (b) Lateral decubitus abdominal X-ray demonstrating pneumoperitoneum (arrow).

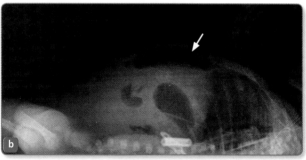

Key facts

- The majority of cases occur due to lymphoid hyperplasia commonly at the ileocaecal valve
- Other causes include Meckel's diverticulum in children of under 3 months of age
- Clinical presentation includes sudden onset abdominal pain, vomiting, 'redcurrant' stools and palpable abdominal mass

- Intussusception can be intermittent with spontaneous resolution

Radiographic findings

US Ultrasound is the modality of choice in diagnosing intussusceptions, evident as a 'target sign' in the transverse plane with a variable number of alternating hyper- and hypoechoic layers (**Figure 10.6a**). This represents the intussusceptum (bowel and mesentery) within the intussuscipiens. In the longitudinal plane the appearance of the intussusceptum is of a 'pseudokidney' (**Figure 10.6b**). Colour Doppler examination of the intussusception is important, as absence of blood flow in the intussusception suggests bowel necrosis.

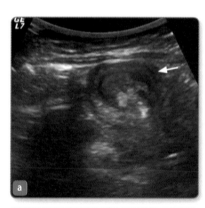

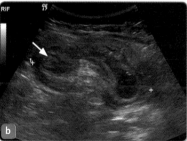

Figure 10.6 (a) Abdominal ultrasound in transverse plane demonstrating a 'target sign' with alternating hyper- and hypoechoic layers (arrow). (b) Abdominal US in the longitudinal plane demonstrating the appearance of a 'pseudokidney' (arrow).

Key signs
- Target sign
- 'Pseudokidney'
- Presence/absence of blood flow in the intussusception

Management
Intussusception can be reduced radiologically by pneumatic reduction. A contraindication for this is pneumoperitoneum, in which case surgery is indicated.

10.3 Musculoskeletal disorders

Fractures
Fracture patterns in children differ from adults due to a decrease in bone mineral density, increased flexibility of the bones, and stronger ligaments and tendons. The epiphyseal plate is a relatively weak point, where fractures are common.

Key facts

Incomplete fractures These do not extend across the bone. Buckle fractures (or torus) result from a bending force that causes the cortex to buckle on the concave side of the fracture (**Figure 10.7**). In greenstick fractures the bone breaks on the convex side of the fracture (**Figure 10.8**). Plastic bowing fractures result in bending/ bowing of the bone with no break in the cortex.

Epiphyseal plate fractures These can vary in severity impacting on both treatment and prognosis with risk of growth disturbance. The Salter Harris classification is used to classify the type of injury from 1 to 5: the higher the grade, the more serious is the injury (**Figure 10.9**). Salter Harris 2 fractures are the most common (**Figure 10.10**).

Avulsion fractures These involve the separation of a fragment of bone at the attachment site of a tendon or ligament. Avulsion of the lesser trochanter is related to an iliopsoas injury (**Figure 10.11**), anterior superior iliac spine with Sartorius injury, anterior inferior iliac spine with rectus femoris injury and adductor avulsion with an inferior ischial ramus injury.

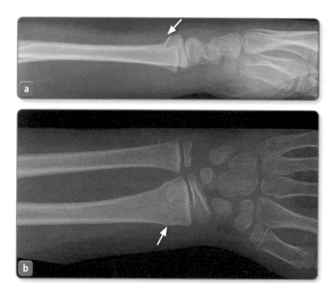

Figure 10.7 (a) Lateral wrist X-ray demonstrating buckle fracture of the distal radius (arrow). (b) Anteroposterior wrist X-ray demonstrating buckle fracture of the distal radius (arrow).

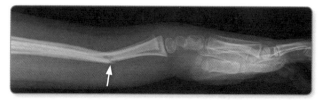

Figure 10.8 Lateral forearm X-ray demonstrating greenstick fractures of the radius and ulna mid shafts (arrow).

Radiographic findings

Plain radiography Plain radiographs are taken in two views at 90 degrees.

Clinical insight

Non-accidental injury usually occurs in children aged <2 years but needs to be considered in all injured children.

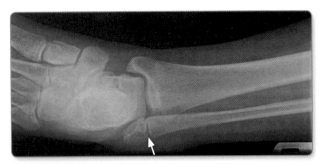

Figure 10.9 Anteroposterior ankle X-ray demonstrating a Salter Harris 1 fracture with widening of the epiphyses of the distal fibula (arrow).

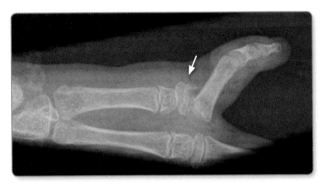

Figure 10.10 Anteroposterior X-ray of left little finger demonstrating a displaced Salter Harris 2 fracture of the proximal phalanx (arrow).

Key signs
- Fracture seen as a break in cortex, lucent line or sclerotic line (bone impacts or overlap)
- Associated dislocation
- Soft tissue swelling/effusion

Management
The management of the fracture will depend on its site, severity of the fracture and associated dislocation.

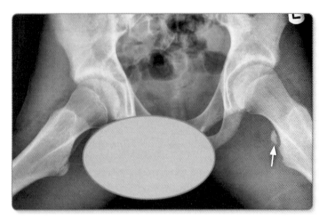

Figure 10.11 Anteroposterior frog-leg X-ray of the pelvis demonstrating an avulsion fracture of the left lesser tronchanter (arrow).

Slipped upper femoral epiphyses

Slipped upper femoral epiphyses (SUFE) is a Salter Harris type 1 fracture involving the femoral epiphyses. SUFE occurs in ages 10–15 years with predisposing factors that include obesity, rickets, endocrine therapy and renal osteodystrophy.

Key facts

- SUFE can be bilateral
- Common in males
- Child may present with hip pain or knee pain
- Complications of SUFE include avascular necrosis of the femoral head, femoral head deformity, osteoarthritis and early closure of growth plate resulting in limb length discrepancy

Radiographic findings

Plain radiography An anteroposterior (AP) pelvic X-ray and a frog lateral X-ray are performed. In the pre slip phase there is a widening of the epiphyseal growth plate. The growth plate is irregular and blurred. In the acute phase the growth plate is displaced posteromedially and may appear smaller due to the posterior slip (**Figure 10.12**). A line drawn along the superior edge of the femoral neck normally intersects the femoral head (line of Klein). In SUFE, the line fails to intersect the femoral head. In a chronic slip, there is sclerosis and irregularity of the growth plate.

Key signs
- Growth plate appears smaller
- Irregularity and blurring of the growth plate
- Line of Klein fails to intersect the femoral head

Management
Management of SUFE includes pinning of the femoral head.

Osteonecrosis of the femoral head
The femoral head is a common site of idiopathic avascular necrosis in children. This is caused by insufficient blood supply to the growth plate.

Key facts
- Commonly occurs from age 3–12 years with patient presenting with hip pain

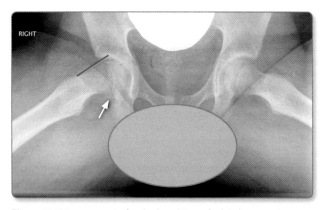

Figure 10.12 Anteroposterior frog-leg lateral X-ray of pelvis demonstrating a right slipped upper femoral epiphyses (arrow). The line of Klein fails to intersect the right femoral head (blue line).

- Can be bilateral
- Although mostly idiopathic, avascular necrosis can be a complication of trauma (SUFE)

Radiographic findings

Plain radiography An AP pelvis X-ray and a frog lateral X-ray are performed. Early radiographic signs include a smaller femoral epiphyses, sclerosis and osteopenia. Late radiographic signs include subchondral fractures of the anterior articular surface (**Figure 10.13**) and fragmentation of the femoral head.

Key signs

- Normal X-ray
- Smaller femoral epiphyses
- Sclerosis of femoral epiphyses
- Subchondral fracture and fragmentation

Management

Management depends on the severity of the osteonecrosis and can be conservative or operative.

> **Clinical insight**
>
> Painful hip is a common clinical presentation. The differential diagnosis can be narrowed by patient's age and clinical history. Differentials include transient synovitis, septic arthritis, osteomyelitis, SUFE, osteonecrosis and avulsion fractures.

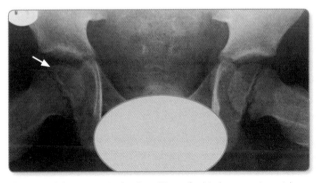

Figure 10.13 Anteroposterior frog lateral X-ray of pelvis demonstrating a right subchondral fracture of the femoral head (arrow).

Index

Note: Page numbers in **bold** or *italic* refer to tables or figures respectively.